Atlas *of* Fetal and Postnatal Brain MR

Paul D. Griffiths, PhD, FRCR
Professor of Radiology and Head of Department, Academic Unit of Radiology,
University of Sheffield, Sheffield, United Kingdom

Janet Morris, MSc
Senior Radiographer, University of Sheffield, Sheffield, United Kingdom

Jeanne-Claudie Larroche
Ex-Directeur de Recherches au CNRS, Hôpital Port-Royal, Paris, France

Michael Reeves, FRCR
Clinical Research Fellow, Academic Unit of Radiology, University of Sheffield, Sheffield,
United Kingdom

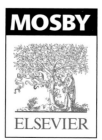

MOSBY

ELSEVIER

1600 John F. Kennedy Blvd.
Ste 1800
Philadelphia, PA 19103-2899

ATLAS OF FETAL AND POSTNATAL BRAIN MR   ISBN: 978-0-323-05296-2

Library of Congress Cataloging-in-Publication Data

Atlas of fetal and postnatal brain MR / Paul D. Griffiths — [et al.]. — 1st ed.
  p. ; cm.
  Includes bibliographical references and index.
  ISBN 978-0-323-05296-2
  1. Fetal brain—Magnetic resonance imaging—Atlases. 2. Newborn infants—Diseases—Diagnosis—Atlases. 3. Developmental neurology—Atlases. 4. Pediatric neurology—Atlases.
I. Griffiths, Paul, 1960 Feb. 27-
  [DNLM: 1. Brain—anatomy & histology—Atlases. 2. Fetus. 3. Infant. 4. Magnetic Resonance Imaging—Atlases. WL 17 A88345 2009]
  RG629.B73A86 2009
  618.92'01—dc22

                                                 2009039290

Acquisitions Editor: Rebecca Gaertner
Editorial Assistant: David Mack
Project Manager: David Saltzberg
Design Direction: Steve Stave

Printed in the United States of America

Last digit is the print number: 9 8 7 6 5 4 3 2 1

It became obvious in the late 1990s that magnetic resonance (MR) imaging of the fetal central nervous system was going to be more than an intellectual curiosity wrapped around a technical challenge. There was (and remains in some circles) some resistance to accept that there is any need for supplementing ultrasonography with fetal MR in cases of suspected developmental brain abnormalities. Many recent studies have shown value of in utero MR of the fetus and there is also gathering interest in postmortem MR of the fetus as an adjunct or replacement to autopsy. The problem was how to start. Few radiologists have experience of the normal MR appearances of the brain at 20 to 40 weeks gestational age. Those who do have the experience have usually gained it from imaging premature babies in whom the predominant pathologies are the complications of prematurity, not malformations. It has taken us a long time to build up a base of normal fetal brain examinations; therefore our appreciation of age-related normality was slow to form. We hope, therefore, that this atlas will help others in this complex area of image interpretation. We must accept that fetal MR (particularly in utero MR) is still in its early stages of development. It is likely that in a few years I will look back in horror at the quality of the images that we were expected to interpret, very much like modern feto-maternal experts reviewing early obstetric ultrasonography. But you have to start somewhere.

When I was struggling to come to terms with mid-trimester brain anatomy I was fortunate to be directed to the pathology atlas of Alison Fess-Higgins and Jeanne-Claudie Larroche. The book was out of print and proved difficult to find but once it was located it was invaluable. It occurred to me first of all that the book should be reprinted, but then considered an updated work including MR. I managed to contact Professor Larroche and was very pleased when she agreed to co-author this updated work with the Sheffield group. It has been a great privilege to work with her.

On a personal level, I have to mention my wife Jane, who is my inspiration, and on occasion, my refuge. Professionally, I would like to acknowledge a number of people who have influenced me over the years. Some have shaped my thinking by reading their papers, hearing them lecture, and subsequently coming to think of them as colleagues and I would include Jim Barkovich, Tom Naidich, Susan Blaser, and Erin Simon in that group. More fundamentally, however, I need to acknowledge the great burden of gratitude I owe to two people who shaped my career at different stages. First, Professor Ian Isherwood, Professor of Radiology at the University of Manchester, who persuaded me to become a neuroradiologist sometime in 1987, having known very little about the speciality previously. And then there was the late Derek Harwood-Nash! It was during my period at the Hospital for Sick Children, Toronto, as the Neuroradiology scholar in 1994-95 that Derek convinced me that pediatric neuroradiology was the only game in town, a decision I have not regretted since!

Paul D. Griffiths

When people listen to you don't you know it means a lot?
'Cause you've got to work so hard for everything you've got
Can't rest on your laurels now not when you've got none
You'll find yourself in a gutter right back where you came from.

Novelty (I. Curtis)

contents

INTRODUCTION

The development of the brain is an exceptionally complicated process, which makes interpretation of radiologic images of the fetal brain challenging. Imaging of the immature brain has become important in recent years for several reasons, with a corresponding increased requirement for clinicians with experience in fetal and neonatal brain imaging. One reason for this need is the desire to detect abnormalities of the brain during the second trimester of pregnancy in order to provide the best-quality information to parents about the likely clinical sequelae of the anomaly. Second is the need to investigate the increasing number of neonates surviving premature delivery who are at high risk for intracranial complications, both hemorrhagic and hypoxic/ischemic. The need for imaging and the manner in which it is delivered has influenced the techniques used. One of the overriding requirements is to not expose the fetus or child to ionizing radiation or at least to keep the exposure to the barest minimum because the potential risks are high in this population. A screening program of second-trimester fetuses cannot be built around an X-ray–based technique such as X-ray computed tomography (CT), hence the rapid rise and refinement of antenatal ultrasonography over the last few decades. It is also desirable to limit the amount of X-rays to which newborn babies are exposed, and ultrasonography has an important role here as well, although other factors are at play. Some ultrasound machines are relatively inexpensive and are portable, making them ideal for use in neonatal intensive care units given the risk management issues associated with moving a child from the neonatal intensive care unit to the radiology department.

Recent studies have shown the limitations of ultrasound for assessment of the fetal and neonatal brain that make the diagnosis of some types of pathology difficult or impossible. For example, the early stages of neonatal hypoxic/ischemic brain injury are difficult to show with transfontanelle ultrasonography; they are shown much better by X-ray CT or magnetic resonance (MR) imaging, particularly using diffusion-weighted imaging. It is becoming increasingly apparent that in utero detection of some developmental brain abnormalities is difficult with ultrasound; agenesis of the corpus callosum is a leading example. These factors have led many groups to explore alternative methods of fetal and neonatal neuroimaging, most of which involve MR imaging. Another use for MR imaging of the immature brain that has been explored by a small number of groups, including our own, is postmortem MR imaging as either an adjunct or an alternative to autopsy. The drive for this in the United Kingdom is the reduction in uptake of fetal/neonatal autopsy by parents concerned about the well-publicized retention of tissues and organs without consent at some British hospitals. It is possible to gain valuable information about brain abnormalities in the post 16-week fetus using postmortem MR imaging and to inform parents about the risk to future pregnancies based on the anatomic definition of the malformation.

The requirements for MR imaging of the brain in these three situations (in utero, postmortem, and postnatal) are fundamentally different, but all have been made possible by significant technologic advances in the field. They are also linked by another factor, namely, problems in interpretation for the reporter. A clinician who reports imaging studies from any specialty has two basic tenets for his/her work: knowledge of normality and knowledge of pathology. The purpose of this book is to assist clinical personnel involved in providing an imaging service to learn and understand normal MR appearances of the brain from the second half of pregnancy to 18 months postnatally.

The histologic basis of this book is the *Development of the Human Foetal Brain: An Anatomical Atlas* by Feess-Higgins and Larroche,[1] which was published in the 1980s but has been out of print for some time. It has been a great privilege for us to work with Professor Larroche on this project. We have used a large number of the line diagrams and histologic photographs from the original INSERM publication in the production of this atlas. The text of the original publication was in French and in English. The annotation of the line diagrams was in Latin, as was the classic approach. We have decided to use a more anglicized approach to the anatomic descriptions, more often than not using the nomenclature provided by Carpenter's *Core Text of Neuroanatomy.*[2]

One of the primary goals of this atlas is to assist doctors who report brain imaging in interpreting in utero MR (iuMR) examinations, a procedure that is gaining in popularity as many centers begin to offer a fetal MR service. MR imaging of the fetus is not recommended before 19 weeks' gestational age (calculated from last menstrual period, as are all of the dates in this book); therefore we start our imaging at 19 to 20 weeks' gestational age. From that maturity to 37 weeks, we present iuMR and postmortem MR (pmMR) images to match the histologic sections and line diagrams as closely as possible. This atlas is illustrated with T2-weighted MR imaging only in fetuses for reasons that are outlined later in the book. Unlike the original Larroche atlas, we continue into the postnatal period, showing both T1- and T2-weighted images of normal infants up to 18 months.

OVERALL LAYOUT OF THE ATLAS

As explained previously, the core of this atlas is the histologic sections and line diagrams published by Professor Larroche more than 20 years ago. The first section of this atlas merely reproduces the images of surface views of the fetal brain, but we use only the gestational ages shown in cross-sectional detail in Section 2. We do not show fetuses ranging from 10 to 18 weeks' gestational age that were included in the original atlas because we do not perform iuMR imaging at those early ages. The images of the surface anatomy of the brains are included to highlight the huge changes occurring in the late second- and third-trimester brain, particularly with respect to sulcation of the cerebral hemispheres. We go into some detail about the timing of the appearance of the major sulci at the start of Section 1 and give an overview about the appearance of sulci in the "mature" brain.

Section 2 shows images from six sequential gestational age periods ranging from 19 to 37 weeks and shows pmMR and iuMR images matched as closely as possible to the tissue sections and line diagrams of the original atlas. One of the most important features of fetal brains during that period is the complicated appearance of transient structures within the developing cerebral wall. We provide a simplified overview of those structures with the aim of assisting interpretation of fetal MR images.

Section 3 shows images of the brain from infants after birth for whom iuMR imaging is not a consideration. Six ages (ranges) are illustrated: 0 to 1 month, 3 to 4 months, 6 months, 9 months, 12 months, and 18 months. For all of the cases we provide the appropriate line diagram of anatomic features from the 40-week fetus of the Larroche atlas. The primary purpose of doing so is to remind the reader of the importance not only of knowing the gross anatomy of the brain but of becoming familiar with the normal patterns of myelination.

DESCRIPTIONS OF THE TECHNIQUES USED

We use four different methods to show the neuroanatomy of the fetus and infant in this atlas: postmortem tissue sections, pmMR, iuMR, and postnatal MR imaging of live children. The techniques used for each of the methods are described here.

Postmortem Fetal Tissue Sections

Brains that appeared normal were chosen for the study. Cases were excluded if the pregnancy was complicated by maternal diabetes, toxemia, intrauterine growth restriction, viral or parasitic fetal infection, maternofetal bacterial infection, or blood group incompatibility. Brains with malformations were excluded, as were cases with large hemorrhages that altered the appearance of the brain. Most of the cases were infants who were stillborn or who survived for only a few hours or days. Exceptionally, survival for 10 days and 2 weeks has been accepted and the corrected age calculated (gestational age plus survival time). The brains were weighed in the fresh state, but because fetal brain tissue is extremely fragile the brains were fixed in formalin before being measured and photographed. After dehydration the brains were embedded whole in celloidin and cut in serial sections at 30 μm. (Techniques for obtaining postmortem fetal tissue sections are modified from Feess-Higgins and Larroche.[1])

The histologic stains used were hematoxylin–eosin, cresyl violet, and the myelin stains Loyez and Luxol fast blue.

Postmortem MR Imaging of the Fetus

The rationale behind our program of pmMR imaging of the fetal central nervous system was to explore the possibility of using imaging as either an adjunct or an alternative to autopsy. The interested reader is directed to some of our earlier publications.[3–5] The majority of our cases resulted from either therapeutic abortions for known central nervous system abnormalities shown on antenatal sonography or from spontaneous abortions. All of the cases in this book were referred to the pediatric pathology department at Sheffield Children's Hospital, which is a regional referral center for fetal and pediatric autopsies. The parents were asked to consent to MR imaging as well as the formal autopsy. All of the pmMR cases shown in this atlas had no abnormality of any description shown on autopsy, pmMR imaging, or any chromosomal/genetic tests performed subsequently.

MR imaging is exquisitely sensitive to patient movement, which usually imposes limits on image acquisition time. This is not an issue when imaging postmortem, and long acquisitions with improved signal-to-noise ratios can be obtained. We took full advantage of this in our earlier cases, routinely acquiring four excitations for each imaging data set. That acquisition required more than 12 minutes for each T2-weighted sequence at 1.5 T, but we subsequently dropped to two excitations at 6 minutes with little noticeable reduction in image quality.

The fundamental goal of this type of imaging is to obtain images with the highest anatomic resolution possible (defined as the smallest objects that can be resolved as separate). The two key elements in providing anatomic resolution are spatial resolution and contrast resolution. Spatial resolution in imaging is dependent on the field of view and matrix size if the amount of MR signal is not otherwise limited. Contrast resolution is the ability to distinguish between two adjacent tissues of different composition. In MR imaging this can be optimized by knowing the composition of the tissue of interest and modifying the MR sequences accordingly. In this respect, MR imaging and X-ray CT have comparable in-plane anatomic resolution, but the improved contrast resolution of brain structures provided by MR imaging makes it the method of choice in most circumstances.

The choice of sequence parameters is important for pmMR imaging. Over the 8 years that we have performed pmMR, we have concluded that the best anatomic information from unfixed brain comes from T2-weighted images. As described in detail in Section 2, this is in contrast to other groups that studied fixed fetal brains. In that situation, T1-weighted images seem optimal, at least in second-trimester fetuses. The precise optimal parameters we use for T2-weighted images required lengthy empirical experimentation (i.e., inspired guesswork!) in earlier pilot studies, but there were theoretical and observational reasons to believe that T2-weighted images would be superior. This is in comparison with imaging of the adult brain, in which gray matter and white matter are best resolved on T1-weighted images. This can be explained by knowledge of the chemical differences between the brains of fetuses and adults/older children. MR images rely on hydrogen nuclei, and the most abundant forms in the body are water and lipids. There is approximately 82% water in mature gray matter and 72% water in myelinated white matter,[6] and more lipid is present in myelinated white matter than in gray matter (54.9% dry weight vs 32.7%[7]). These two factors account for the superb gray/white distinction on T1-weighted MR imaging, particularly on T1 in the fully myelinated brain. The major difference in the brains of fetuses compared to adult brains is the virtual absence of myelin. In this case, the water content and the lipid content of gray and "white" matter in the fetus are similar, leading to the prediction of poor tissue contrast. This certainly is the case for T1-weighted images where even in the "ideal" imaging conditions of pmMR, obtaining a T1 sequence with good tissue contrast for normal brain structures at 1.5 T is difficult, at least in our experience. Tissue contrast between the future gray matter and white matter structures is present on T2-weighted sequences, but the contrast is modest. However, some structures present in the fetal brain, such as neuronal and glial periventricular formation areas (germinal matrix) and the "transient fetal zones" within the developing cerebral hemispheres as described, greatly improve the predicted tissue contrast resolution.

The examinations shown in this atlas were performed using either a 1.5-T or 3-T superconducting system (Infinion 1.5T or Intera 3.0T, Philips Medical Systems, Best, Netherlands). Brain imaging consisted of high-resolution imaging in the three orthogonal planes using fast spin echo methods to produce T2-weighted images using either a wrist or a knee coil (depending on the size of the fetus). The sequences at 1.5 T consisted of fast spin echo (echo train length 32) T2-weighted images (TR 15,662 ms, TE 92 ms) with a bandwidth of 20.8 kHz using two acquisitions. A field of view of 14 cm and matrix size of 256 × 256 were used, giving in-plane resolution of 0.5-mm and 2-mm thick slices (no interslice gap) of the whole brain. These parameters have now been used extensively to show both developmental and acquired fetal brain pathology postmortem (Figure 1).

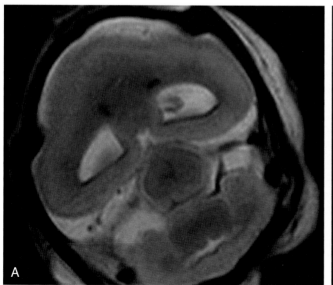 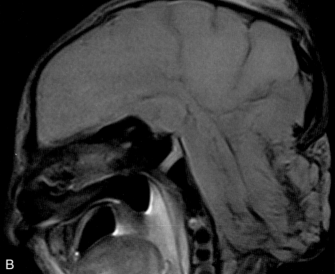

Figure 1   Postmortem magnetic resonance imaging at 1.5 T from two different cases. **A,** Image of an early second-trimester fetus with alobar holoprosencephaly. **B,** Sagittal image of an early third-trimester fetus with a low occipital encephalocoele extending into the upper cervical region.

The cases included in this atlas acquired after 2006 were taken on a 3-T system. In theory, imaging at higher field strength should improve both anatomic and tissue resolution of the fetal brain and allow better delineation of the complicated infrastructure of the developing brain. Anecdotally this appears to be correct, but formal comparison is pending. The sequence data at 3 T are fast spin echo T2-weighted, echo train length 10, TR 4000 ms, TE 200 ms, flip angle 90°, field of view 120 mm, with reconstructed matrix size 640 × 640. Thirty 2-mm-thick slices with no gap and two excitations take 16 minutes to acquire. The resulting images produce excellent delineation of normal and abnormal fetal brain anatomy, but we also obtained some early good results producing T1-weighted images at 3 T (Figure 2).

In Utero MR Imaging of the Fetus

Our group has performed iuMR studies of the fetal brain since 1999 when clinical MR scanners with sufficient gradient power to perform ultrafast imaging were being produced. Fetal MR imaging had been performed before that time, but mechanisms for preventing the fetus from moving were needed. Some groups used muscular blockade of the fetus with pancuronium administration into the umbilical vessels, usually while the vessel was being cannulated for another reason. Good images were obtained using standard sequences, but the procedure was highly invasive and was associated with risk to the fetus. A less invasive approach used intravenous benzodiazepines to sedate the fetus, but monitoring the mother in the MR environment presented other problems. The introduction of ultrafast MR imaging methods into clinical practice has made iuMR imaging (potentially) widely accessible.

Our approach to iuMR imaging has been published previously,[8] as have our results showing many advantages of iuMR imaging over ultrasonography for developmental fetal neuropathology.[9,10] One of the problems we faced was lack of knowledge of normal second-trimester fetal anatomy as demonstrated by MR imaging. This problem continued for a considerable time because our examinations for the first 4 years were performed as research studies. We did not have approval from our local research ethics committee to study women with normal pregnancies because of the unknown effects of iuMR imaging on the fetus, so we investigated only those fetuses with known or suspected abnormality on ultrasonography. This is still the case now, although we offered fetomaternal and genetic centers an iuMR facility (with the support of our local research ethics committee) to study women whose fetus was at higher risk from brain and/or spine malformation. Many of those fetuses were normal, and by obtaining clinical follow-up of those children, we built up a library of normal cases, some of which are used to illustrate this book.

Full written consent is obtained from the woman by the attending radiologist after explanation of the procedure. She is screened for the known contraindications to MR, as is her partner or relative if he/she intends to go into the MR scanner room with the mother. A flexible phased-array coil is placed around the lower abdomen, and a series of three plane scout views is made to locate the fetal brain. Fetal imaging is first performed in an attempt to image the brain in the three natural orthogonal planes using single-shot fast spin echo (SSFSE) sequences initially with 5-mm-thick sections. The sequence parameters are TR 20,000 ms, TE 93.6 ms, field of view 250 mm, matrix size 232 × 256, echo train length 128, and flip angle 90°. The studies then are repeated using 3-mm-thick sections with parameters TR 21,032 ms, TE 103.6 ms, field of view 250 mm, matrix size 256 × 256, echo train length 140, and flip angle 90°. The acquisition times typically are 20 and

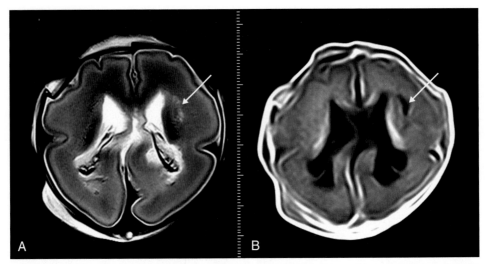

Figure 2 Axial images at 3.0 T from postmortem magnetic resonance examination of a fetus with ventriculomegaly and hypoplasia of the corpus callosum (confirmed on sagittal imaging). **A,** Routine T2-weighted image. **B,** Equivalent T1-weighted image. Note the high-signal germinal matrix and cortical plate on the T1 image. This contrast is a great improvement over the 1.5-T imaging we performed earlier. Note that the region superficial to the left germinal matrix shows postmortem damage and artifactual signal disturbance.

25 seconds, respectively. These sequences provide heavily T2-weighted images. As part of our imaging protocol, we also acquire T1-weighted images in at least one plane (usually axial). The sequence we currently use is T1 RFFAST with parameters TR 210 ms, TE 4.47 ms, flip angle 80°, bandwidth 41.67 kHz, field of view 250 mm, and matrix size 256×140. Twenty 5-mm-thick sections take 29 seconds to acquire.

The major problem with T1-weighted iuMR images of the fetal brain is the lack of inherent tissue contrast because of high water and low lipid content. This combination produces a very "flat" image that, in our experience, has poor delineation even of the normal high signal from the germinal matrices on T1-weighted images. Therefore we use this sequence to look for abnormal fat-containing structures or subacute hemorrhage. No T1-weighted fetal images are shown in this atlas. Although the individual acquisitions are only in the order of 20 to 30 seconds, the table occupancy time can be quite long because of fetal movement and the "chasing" required to obtain the orthogonal planes. Experienced radiographers are vital to reduce the overall examination time; in most cases we can obtain all of the sequences described in less than 20 minutes.

Postnatal MR Imaging

The five cases used to illustrate the postnatal section are taken from children who were being investigated for possible head injuries but who had no focal neurologic problems, had normal X-ray CT and MR examinations, and were normal at clinical follow-up. All of the children were examined under general anesthesia using the following parameters: (1) Fast spin echo T2-weighted, echo train length 8, TR 4500 ms, TE 94.5 ms, field of view 240 mm, matrix size 352×512, two excitations. Sections 5 mm thick were taken with a 1-mm gap, and 21 slices took 6 minutes 36 seconds to acquire. (2) Spin echo T1-weighted, TR 588 ms, TE 15.2 ms, field of view 240 mm, matrix size 256×256, two excitations. Sections 5 mm thick were taken with a 1-mm gap, and 21 slices took 5 minutes 2 seconds to acquire.

Differences Between the Techniques

The three imaging methods used to illustrate fetal brain anatomy in this atlas are not directly comparable for many reasons. The first and most obvious problem is that the iuMR, pmMR, and histologic sections were obtained from different individuals. Sufficient variation among individual fetal brains ensures that perfect matches can never be made. An added complication arises when trying to ensure the sections have been taken from matched anatomic planes. This is a particular problem for axial and coronal images where the planes of section are arbitrary, unlike sagittal/parasagittal images where the plane of section is easily defined. We use the tissue sections in the original Larroche atlas as the reference

standard in this book and attempt to match the MR images to the tissue sections. This is relatively easy with pmMR imaging because scan time is not an issue and there are no problems with movement. In contrast, this is a major problem for iuMR because of the small moving target and the limited amount of time we believe a pregnant woman should be kept on the MR scanner.

There are, however, more fundamental differences between the methods. The fetal tissue sections used in the study came from brains that had been removed from the calvarium and fixed prior to staining. This has certain obvious and inevitable consequences. First, a large proportion of the extraaxial anatomy is lost, unlike the in situ pmMR cases shown in this atlas and the iuMR cases. Second, the fixation process itself likely has some effect on the overall morphology of the brain as the alteration of protein elements and the removal of water likely have differential effects on different parts of the brain. For example, in our experience (and that of other workers), the cortical sulci appear more prominent on tissue sections than on pmMR images when fetuses of the same gestational age are matched. It also is likely that the relative effacement of cortical sulci seen on pmMR imaging compared to the other techniques results from premortem swelling of the brain prior to abortion.

One of the major advantages of histologic studies of the brain is the ability to use different staining methods to show different cellular elements to advantage. The two categories of stains used in the Larroche atlas were "histologic" (hematoxylin–eosin or cresyl violet) and myelin stains (Loyez or Luxol fast blue). Although we can use different sequences and parameters in pmMR imaging, we cannot hope to rival the tissue contrast provided by histologic stains. In some cases this is of little detriment; for example, the germinal matrix has a significantly lower signal on T2-weighted images and is well demonstrated on both pmMR images and stained tissue sections. On the other hand, the transient layers within the fetal white matter are present but are more difficult to separate on pmMR images than on histologic sections. It should also be remembered that MR sections are much thicker than histologic sections.

Many other features seen in postmortem fetal brains result either from the effects of the fetal demise itself or as a complication of traumatic delivery. Some damage to normal brain anatomy is commonly seen on postmortem studies (both autopsy and pmMR), and some structures (e.g., fetal corpus callosum) show marked susceptibility to artifactual injury. This was discussed in Larroche's atlas and is seen on pmMR, such as the 19- to 20-week case used to illustrate this book. MR imaging is highly sensitive to early subacute hemorrhage, and intraventricular, germinal matrix, and/or choroid plexus hemorrhage are commonly seen on postmortem MR. We believe that, in many cases, this is an effect of the fetal loss per se and is not the cause of the abortion.

There are also major differences between postmortem and in utero fetal imaging studies. The SSFSE T2-weighted images used to acquire rapid images of the fetus do not allow great definition of the ultrastructure of the developing cerebral hemispheres. The germinal matrix often can be distinguished in the second-trimester fetus, but the transient layers frequently are indistinct. Another significant difference between iuMR, pmMR, and tissue sections are the sizes of the extraaxial spaces and ventricles. The ventricles look smaller on tissue sections than on iuMR images and look considerably smaller on pmMR images. The size of the extra-axial cerebrospinal fluid spaces can be compared on iuMR and pmMR images (where the brain is still in situ), and in many cases the subarachnoid space is barely seen on pmMR images but is very prominent on iuMR images. This is almost certainly due to lack of cerebrospinal fluid after fetal demise, perhaps combined with premortem swelling of the fetal brain prior to abortion. One other effect of this difference is that the cortical sulci that have formed appear more prominent on iuMR, although the degree of sulcation is no different.

In spite of these differences, the wealth of anatomic knowledge amassed from the study of histologic sections over the years can be used to assist with the interpretation of pmMR and iuMR examinations.

REFERENCES

1. Feess-Higgins A, Larroche J-C: In Feess-Higgins A, Larroche J-C (eds): Development of the Human Foetal Brain: An Anatomical Atlas. Paris, INSERM CNRS, 1987, pp 13–189.
2. Carpenter MB: Core Text of Neuroanatomy, 4th ed. Baltimore, Williams & Wilkins, 1991.
3. Griffiths PD, Variend D, Evans M, et al: Post mortem magnetic resonance imaging of the fetal and stillborn central nervous system. Am J Neuroradiol 24:22–27, 2003.
4. Griffiths PD, Paley MNJ, Whitby EH: Post-mortem MR imaging as an alternative to fetal/neonatal autopsy: The position in 2005. Lancet 365:1271–1273, 2005.
5. Widjaja E, Whitby EH, Paley MNJ, Griffiths PD: Normal fetal lumbar spine on post-mortem MR imaging. Am J Neuroradiol 27:553–559, 2006.
6. Van der Knaap MS, Valk J: Myelin and white matter. In Van der Knaap MS, Valk J (eds): Magnetic Resonance of Myelin, Myelination and Myelin Disorders, 2nd ed. Berlin, Springer, 1995, pp 1–17.
7. Norton WT, Cammer W: Isolation and characterization of myelin. In Morrel P (ed): Myelin. New York, Plenum, 1984, pp 147–195.
8. Griffiths PD, Paley MNJ, Widjaja E, Taylor C, Whitby EH: The emergence of in utero MR imaging for fetal brain and spine abnormalities. BMJ 331:562–565, 2005.
9. Whitby EH, Paley MNJ, Sprigg A, et al: Outcome of 100 singleton pregnancies with suspected brain abnormalities diagnosed on ultrasound and investigated by in utero MR imaging. Br J Obstet Gynaecol 111:784–792, 2004.
10. Griffiths PD, Widjaja E, Paley MNJ, Whitby EH: Imaging the fetal spine using in utero MR: Diagnostic accuracy and impact on management. Pediatr Radiol 36:927–933, 2006.

SURFACE ANATOMY OF THE BRAIN

The adult human brain has a highly complex external morphology, and this is particularly true of the cerebral hemispheres. The clinical neuroimager needs to know the normal patterns of cortical gyri and their associated sulci in order to make accurate anatomic diagnoses that will assist in functional assessment and/or surgical planning. Someone looking at the surface of the adult brain for the first time likely would be convinced by the apparent randomness of the convoluted surface. However, it becomes apparent that the gyri/sulci form patterns that are common among individuals and, although variations exist, a large number of recurring themes can be found. It is important for anyone trying to understand the development of fetal cerebral hemispheres for diagnostic purposes to have a deep understanding of the final adult patterns and common variations. It is also necessary to appreciate the gestalt of being able to understand the surface anatomy of the brain and applying that knowledge when interpreting cross-sectional imaging studies. Naidich et al.[1,2] have provided many illuminating publications on the subject, and the interested reader is directed to their work.

Before 16 weeks' gestational age the fetal human cerebral hemispheres are effectively smooth and featureless. In contrast, the overall degree of sulcation at birth is effectively the same as the adult pattern. The huge changes in the external morphology of the brain that occur between those two time points are due to the development of the cerebral cortex and the massive numbers of neurons and glia that migrate there from the germinal matrices. The gyral convolutions produce a greater surface area per unit volume compared with the smooth, agyric cortex present in many other mammals. Indeed, the gyric human cerebral cortex is estimated to have three times the surface area as an agyric brain of the same volume. The major sulci of the brain tend to appear in an ordered and predictable sequence, and the person interpreting fetal magnetic resonance (MR) images should be aware of the normal patterns and schedules of appearance. However, the patterns are only approximations, and one should not expect to be able to define with any degree of accuracy the gestational age of a fetus based on the sulcal patterns. Biologic variation is one issue, and the mechanisms for estimating the dates of a pregnancy have wide margins of error. In addition, the possible significant differences in the degree of sulcation between the two hemispheres within the same individual are well documented.

The purpose of this section is to show the development of the surface cortical patterns of the fetal brain between 19 weeks' gestational age and term. We recommend that you refer back to this section when studying the cross-sectional images of the appropriate gestational age in Section 2 or the neonatal cases in Section 3 because an understanding of sulcation both on cross-sectional imaging and on representations of surfaces is necessary. This section begins with a discussion of the appearances of the major cortical sulci that may be described as mature" or adult pattern. This section uses the surface projections of the developing fetal brain from the Larroche atlas.[3]

ANATOMY OF THE SULCI AND FISSURES IN THE "MATURE" SUPRATENTORIAL BRAIN

The cerebral hemispheres are separated from each other in the midline by the median (great) longitudinal fissure and its contents: the pia and arachnoid mater with the intervening subarachnoid space that overlie both cerebral hemispheres, and two layers of dura mater that are fused for the most part as the falx cerebri. The inferior sagittal sinus is contained within the free inferior border of the falx, whereas superiorly the two leaves of dura separate to contain the superior sagittal sinus (Figure 1-1). The falx is attached to the crista galli anteriorly, where it is quite narrow, but it widens as it sweeps posteriorly and eventually attaches along the midline of the tentorium cerebelli. The drainage of venous blood in the sagittal sinuses normally is from anterior to posterior; therefore the structure increases in size passing posteriorly to accommodate for increasing drainage from the cortical veins. These features are well shown on coronal MR imaging.

The surfaces of the cerebral hemispheres show many convolutions consisting of cortical gyri separated by

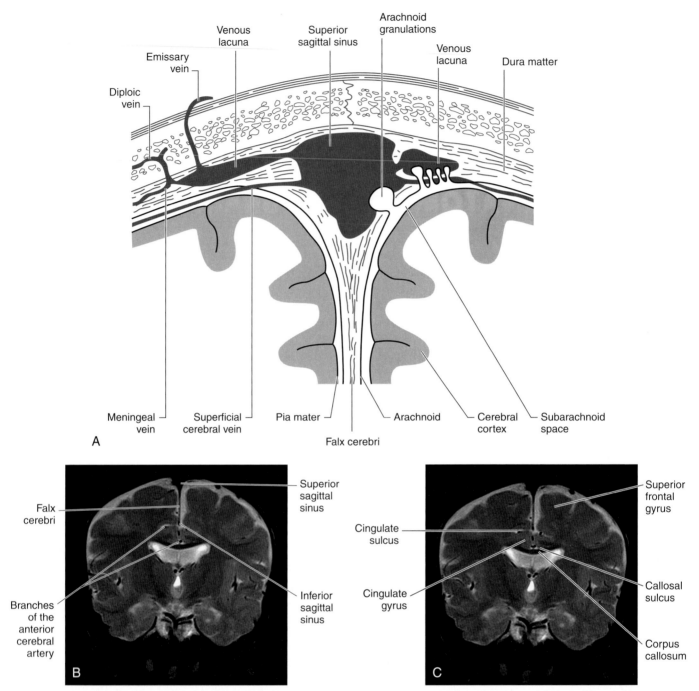

Figure 1-1   Anatomy of the median longitudinal fissure. **A,** Line diagram of the anatomy of the medial longitudinal fissure and its contents in the coronal plane. (From Stranding S [ed]: Gray's Anatomy, 39th ed. Edinburgh, Elsevier, 2005.) **B, C,** Coronal T2-weighted images from a 3-year-old child with mild atrophic changes due to an unknown, progressive degenerative process of the brain. Showing respectively the contents of the median longitudinal fissure and the adjacent brain anatomy. The midline falx cerebri has low signal on this sequence because of its high fibrous content. The superior and inferior sinuses related to either end of the falx have low signal because of flow phenomena (as for the branches of the anterior cerebral artery). Free water has high signal on this sequence, which explains the high signal in the cortical sulci and other cerebrospinal fluid–containing spaces.

sulci of varying sizes. Most of the sulci are prominent and easily delineated in whole brain preparations, and many of them are constant between individuals. The cerebral cortex and associated white matter form four lobes in each hemisphere (frontal, temporal, parietal, occipital), and those lobes are (incompletely) defined by prominent, relatively constant sulci. The appearances of sulci on imaging studies can be appreciated only if the anatomy of the meninges is understood. The innermost layer of the meninges, the pia mater, is closely adherent to the surface of the brain at all sites. In contrast, the thicker arachnoid mater encompasses the brain without extending into the recesses. The subarachnoid space lies between the two, contains cerebrospinal fluid (CSF), and usually is quite thin. However, some regions contain local dilatations of the subarachnoid space with large pools of CSF. One such region is the basal cisterns related to the inferior surface of the brain; another is the space between adjacent cortical gyri. Thus the cortical sulci have the same intensity as the fluid within the ventricles on all sequences (e.g., high signal on T2-weighted images), and their shape is dependent solely on the shape of the adjacent gyri. The major sulci and associated brain structures of a fetus of 40 weeks gestational age are shown in Figure 1-2.

MAJOR SULCI RESPONSIBLE FOR DEFINING LOBAR ANATOMY

These consist of the lateral (sylvian) sulcus, central sulcus, and parieto-occipital sulcus. For the most part the lobar anatomy is best defined on the lateral surface of the brain by the lateral and central sulci.

Lateral Sulcus

The lateral sulcus is a deep fissure that is first identified on the inferior surface of the brain close to the anterior perforated substance but becomes most visible on the lateral surface where it separates the frontal and parietal lobes from the temporal lobe. The frontal lobe is separated completely from the temporal lobe, whereas the posterior aspects of the parietal and temporal lobes remain in continuity without a well-defined external border. The parts of the frontal, temporal, and parietal lobes that protrude into and surround the lateral fissure are called the *opercula*. The anatomy of the lateral sulcus on the lateral surface of the brain is complicated as it divides into three rami: anterior horizontal, anterior ascending, and posterior. These can be seen well on MR imaging that allows nonorthogonal plane reformation of volume data (Figure 1-3). The anterior horizontal ramus protrudes into the inferior frontal gyrus running horizontally and anteriorly. The anterior ascending ramus runs vertically into the same gyrus and defines the pars triangularis portion of the inferior frontal gyrus anterior to the ascending ramus and the pars opercularis posteriorly. The posterior ramus extends posteriorly and slightly superiorly for approximately 8 cm before dividing into the posterior ascending and posterior

descending rami.[4] Naidich et al. have shown that the anatomy of the subcentral gyrus is well seen on MR, and this topic is discussed in the section on locating the central sulcus.

The insula is defined as the cortical surface in the depth of the lateral fissure and is considered to be the "fifth cortical lobe" by some researchers. The mature insula has a complicated surface structure, which is best appreciated on whole brain preparations when the opercula have been removed (similar "virtual" procedures can be performed on T1-weighted volume data; Figure 1-4). The insula is pyramidal in shape, with its apex directed inferiorly and anteriorly. The apex is the only portion of the insula that is not bounded by the circular gyrus. The large central insular sulcus runs from the apex, superiorly and posteriorly to form larger anterior and smaller posterior surfaces. The posterior region usually is divided by a single sulcus to form two "gyri longi," whereas the anterior area is inconsistently divided into three or four "gyri brevi."

Central Sulcus

This prominent sulcus on the lateral aspect of the cerebral hemisphere barely extends onto the medial surface, if at all. The central sulcus separates the frontal and parietal lobes, and the frontal lobe can be completely delineated by the lateral and central sulci on the lateral surface of the brain. It takes a curved course posteriorly at approximately 70° towards the lateral sulcus but does not contact it. The postcentral sulcus lies approximately 1.5 cm posterior to the central sulcus and runs parallel to it. The correct localization of the central sulcus is hugely important on cross-sectional imaging as it defines the primary motor cortex anteriorly and the primary sensorimotor cortex posteriorly. This can be difficult and is best achieved on axial imaging as described in the section on the cingulate sulcus.

Parieto-occipital Sulcus

This is predominantly a feature of the posterior portion of the medial hemispheric surface, although it can extend onto the lateral surface for a short way in some cases. It runs inferiorly and slightly anteriorly, separating the precuneus of the parietal lobe and the cuneus of the occipital lobe before joining the calcarine fissure.

Note that a temporo-occipital sulcus exists on the inferior surface of the brain but has highly variable appearances.

OTHER SULCI OF IMPORTANCE FOR FETAL IMAGING

Superior and Inferior Frontal Sulci

The lateral surface of the frontal lobe is indented by two sulci running in a broadly horizontal fashion, the superior and inferior frontal sulci. These demarcate

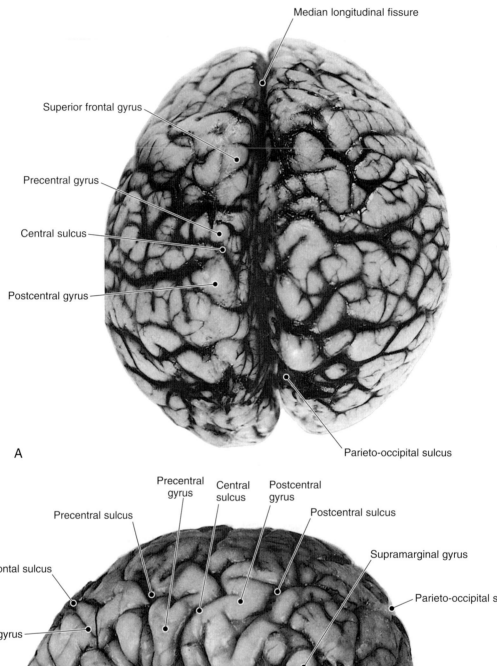

Median longitudinal fissure

Superior frontal gyrus

Precentral gyrus

Central sulcus

Postcentral gyrus

Parieto-occipital sulcus

A

Precentral gyrus

Central sulcus

Postcentral gyrus

Precentral sulcus

Postcentral sulcus

Superior frontal sulcus

Supramarginal gyrus

Parieto-occipital sulcus

Middle frontal gyrus

Inferior frontal gyrus

Occipital lobe

Lateral sulcus

Superior temporal gyrus

Superior temporal sulcus

Inferior temporal sulcus

Middle temporal gyrus

Inferior temporal gyrus

B

Figure 1-2   Surface features of a 40-week gestational age fetus. **A,** Superior. **B,** Lateral.

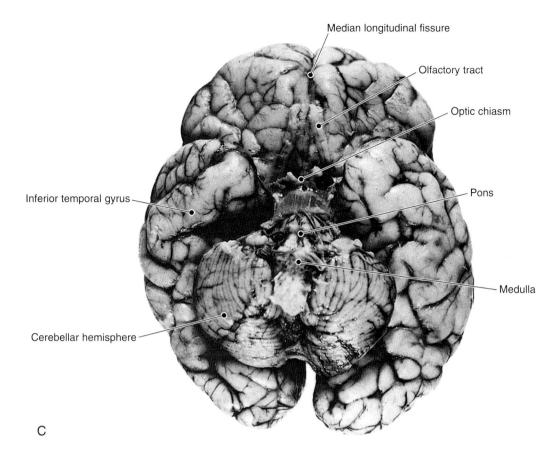

Median longitudinal fissure

Olfactory tract

Optic chiasm

Pons

Inferior temporal gyrus

Medulla

Cerebellar hemisphere

C

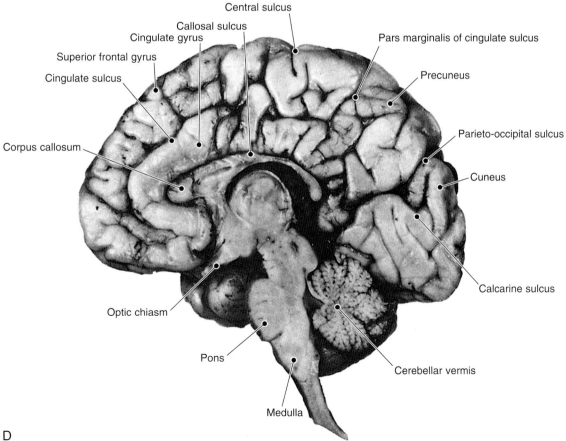

Central sulcus

Callosal sulcus

Cingulate gyrus

Pars marginalis of cingulate sulcus

Superior frontal gyrus

Precuneus

Cingulate sulcus

Parieto-occipital sulcus

Corpus callosum

Cuneus

Optic chiasm

Calcarine sulcus

Pons

Cerebellar vermis

Medulla

D

Figure 1-2, cont'd   **C,** Inferior. **D,** Medial. The same annotation is used for these figures as in the developmental series at the end of the section.

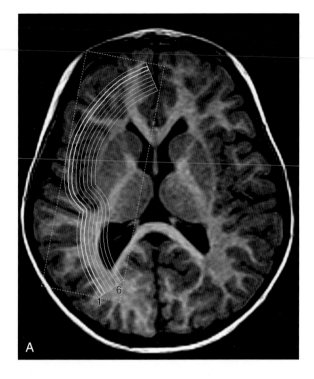

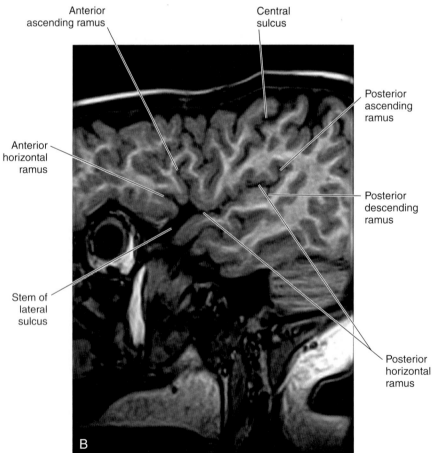

Figure 1-3   Anatomy of the lateral sulcus and surrounding brain on magnetic resonance imaging. The anatomy of the lateral sulcus can be studied on parasagittal sections of the brain but often is best shown using nonorthogonal curvilinear reformations of T1-weighted volume data. **A,** Plane of reformation on axial section (same case as Figure 1-1). **B, C** Same curvilinear reformation showing the sulci and brain structures, respectively. Note the pars orbitalis, pas triangularis, and pars opercularis all are subdivisions of the inferior frontal gyrus.

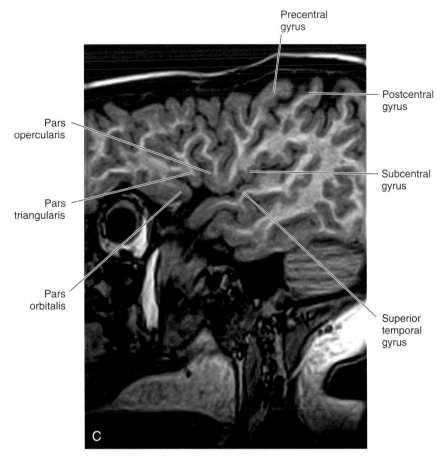

Precentral gyrus

Postcentral gyrus

Pars opercularis

Subcentral gyrus

Pars triangularis

Pars orbitalis

Superior temporal gyrus

C

Figure 1-3, cont'd

the superior frontal gyrus (above the superior frontal sulcus), inferior frontal gyrus (below the inferior frontal sulcus), and middle frontal gyrus between the two. These are well shown on coronal MR images. The precise pattern of sulcation varies a great deal, but most frequently the superior frontal sulcus is deficient posteriorly, allowing continuity between the posterior parts of the superior and middle frontal gyri.

Cingulate Sulcus

The most prominent feature on the medial aspect of the anterior cerebral hemisphere is the cingulate sulcus. The majority of this sulcus is related to the frontal lobe, commencing below the rostrum of the corpus callosum and curving anteriorly and then posteriorly roughly parallel to the corpus callosum and delineating the cingulate gyrus. At a point approximately above the splenium of the corpus callosum, the cingulate sulcus curves upward into the parietal lobe to become the pars marginalis of the cingulate gyrus, which extends onto the superior portion of the lateral aspect of the hemisphere. As described by Naidich et al., this is a useful landmark for locating the central sulcus on cross-sectional imaging.[1]

Superior and Inferior Temporal Sulci

The lateral aspects of the temporal lobes are subdivided in a fashion similar to the frontal lobes. Two horizontally directed sulci, the superior and inferior temporal sulci, divide the surface into three gyri, the superior, middle, and inferior temporal gyri. Posteriorly there exists an indistinct boundary between the temporal gyri and the parietal and occipital lobes.

Calcarine Sulcus

The calcarine sulcus is a feature of the medial surface of the occipital lobe. It is important because the visual cortex lies above and below the calcarine sulcus. It commences at the occipital pole and runs anteriorly to meet the parieto-occipital sulcus.

Collateral Sulcus

The collateral sulcus starts at the occipital pole on the inferior surface of the brain and runs anteriorly parallel to the calcarine sulcus. At its anterior extent it separates the parahippocampal gyrus from the more lateral portions of the temporal lobe. It may join the rhinal sulcus, but more often it remains isolated.

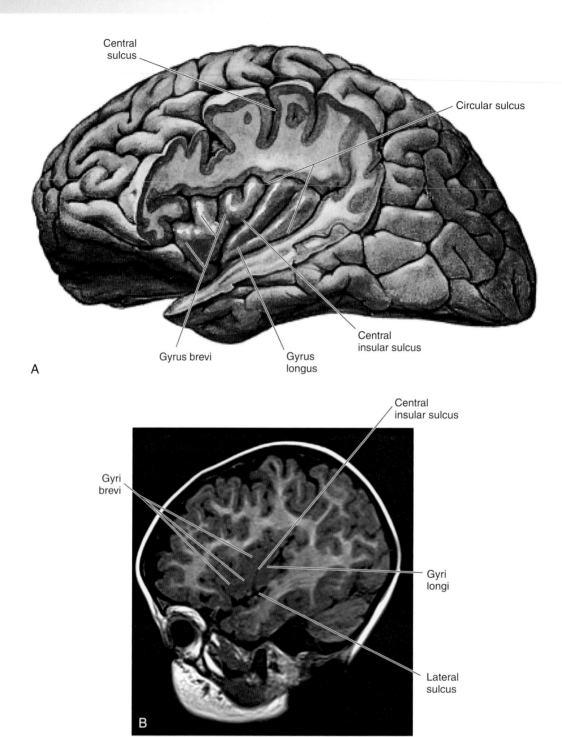

Figure 1-4 Anatomy of the insula. **A,** Line diagram depicting the anatomy of the insula. (From Stranding S [ed]: Gray's Anatomy, 39th ed. Edinburgh, Elsevier, 2005.) **B,** Sagittal oblique reformation of T1-weighted volume images from a child with no structural brain abnormality. The insula is divided into a larger anterior part (containing the gyri brevi) and a smaller posterior part (containing the gyri longi) by the central insular sulcus.

LOCATION OF THE CENTRAL SULCUS ON CROSS-SECTIONAL IMAGING

There are many situations in clinical practice when it is necessary to demonstrate the central sulcus on cross-sectional imaging in order to locate the precentral and postcentral gyri with confidence. This can be done only with an understanding of the anatomy of other sulcal structures. This is best performed on axial imaging for the superior portion of the central sulcus and on parasagittal images for the inferior portion. The anatomy of cortical sulci is best appreciated in older adults in whom some volume loss of the brain results in prominence of the sulci. Conversely, the brains of most children have a relative paucity of CSF-containing structures on the surface, which can make appreciation of sulcal anatomy difficult. Neonates, however, often have prominent sulci (and ventricles), which assists with location of the following structures.

Superior Portion of the Central Sulcus

The key to locating the superior portion of the central sulcus is being able to find the pars marginalis portion of the cingulate sulcus and the postcentral sulcus. As previously described the main stem of the cingulate sulcus is best shown on sagittal imaging just off the midline. The anterior portion of the cingulate sulcus is directly superior to the cingulate gyrus and runs parallel to the corpus callosum. Above the posterior part of the body of the corpus callosum a branch of the cingulate sulcus arcs superiorly. This is the pars marginalis, and it extends onto the superior surface of the cerebral hemispheres for a short distance. As a result, the pars marginalis has a highly characteristic appearance on the superior sections of axial brain images. It appears as an anteriorly curved sulcus that, when both sides are viewed together, has been likened to Salvador Dali's moustache. The position of the pars marginalis in relation to the center of the image is dependent on the angulation of the axial sections. For example, axial MR images usually are set parallel to the anterior/posterior commissural line, which broadly approximates to the plane of the anterior cranial fossa. In this situation the pars marginalis is situated close to the posterior edge of the superior-most axial images (Figure 1-5). If a steeper angulation is made, as for X-ray CT of the brain (in order to reduce radiation dose to the lens of the eyes), the pars marginalis is much closer to the center of the field of view.

In either case the correct location of the pars marginalis must be made by judging its relationship to the postcentral sulcus in the anterior portion of the parietal lobe. The postcentral sulcus appears as a "bracket-shaped" CSF-containing structure that is convex laterally, with neither end of the bracket extending medial to the pars marginalis. In some cases the transverse parietal sulcus contributes to the postcentral "bracket." Once those two structures are located, the central sulcus is easily identified just anterior to the postcentral sulcus. Other features that can confirm the correct anatomy include the following:

- The central sulcus extends medial to and "inside" the curve of the pars marginalis (of the postcentral "bracket," which remains lateral).
- The cortex of the precentral gyrus should be thicker than the cortex of the postcentral gyrus.
- The precentral gyrus has a prominent "knob"-shaped bulge on its posterior aspect that represents the expanded portion of cortex containing the hand motor area.
- More anteriorly, the superior frontal sulcus often joins with the precentral sulcus. It does not join with the central sulcus.

Inferior Portion of the Central Sulcus

Once the central sulcus has been located on the superior-most images, it can be tracked on its pathway inferiorly along the lateral surface of the cerebral hemisphere. However, it is useful to locate the lower portion of the central sulcus on sagittal images, and to do so requires a more detailed review of the anatomy of the lateral sulcus as described by Naidich et al.[5] The posterior horizontal ramus is the longest portion of the lateral sulcus, and it is joined by smaller sulci along its midcourse. Inferiorly, transverse temporal sulci indent the superior temporal gyrus. Of greater importance in locating the central sulcus are the two sulci on the superior aspect of the posterior horizontal ramus: the anterior and posterior subcentral sulci. The small protrusion of the brain between those sulci is the subcentral gyrus, and the central sulcus approaches (but does not contact) the cortex of the gyrus. The precentral gyrus can be located anteriorly and the postcentral gyrus behind (Figure 1-3, *C*).

APPEARANCE OF CORTICAL SULCI ON IN UTERO MR IMAGING IN RELATION TO GESTATIONAL AGE

This subject has been studied in great depth by Dr. Catherine Garel and colleagues, and the reader is directed to her excellent textbook on fetal MR.[6] The cerebral hemispheres separate from each other very early in development, a process that starts in the sixth week of gestation and is complete around 9 to 10 weeks, during a period of intense growth of the cerebral hemispheres termed *ventral and dorsal induction.* The median interhemispheric fissure and falx should be clearly visible in their entirety if fetal imaging is performed at 19 weeks' gestational age or later. Any abnormal communication of forebrain derivatives over the midline defines the group of abnormalities called *holoprosencephaly.*

Sulci Defining Lobar Anatomy

Differences are seen between the conspicuity of cortical sulci on postmortem tissue sections and in utero MR (iuMR) imaging. Specifically, our anecdotal experience indicates delineation of sulci at earlier gestational ages on tissue sections. This is supported by Garel's comparison of her iuMR cases with the pathologic studies of Chi et al.[7] The lateral sulcus is well seen on histologic studies as early as 16 weeks' gestational age but usually is not clearly demarcated in all fetuses at 19 to 20 weeks' gestation. Garel's textbook presents cases at 22 to 23 weeks, and at that stage the lateral sulcus was seen in 100% of normal fetuses. It is not sufficient to know merely when the lateral sulcus can first be located. The lateral sulcus is an exceptionally complicated structure that continues to develop after birth, and an understanding of its normal sequence of development is important. When the lateral sulcus first appears, it is

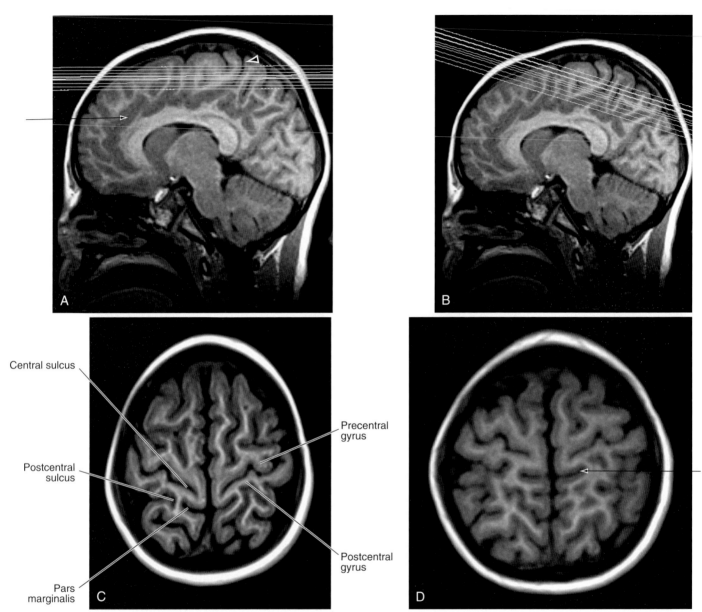

Central sulcus

Precentral gyrus

Postcentral sulcus

Postcentral gyrus

Pars marginalis

Figure 1-5 Effects of scan angulation on the anatomy of the paracentral lobule on axial imaging. All images from a T1-weighted volume data set of a 4-year-old child with no structural brain abnormality. **A,** Sagittal image just off midline showing the cingulate sulcus *(arrow)* and its pars marginalis portion *(arrowhead)*. **B** is the equivalent image showing the approximate angulation used for X-ray computed tomographic procedures. **C** shows the normal anatomy of the paracentral lobule on "MR angulation" whilst **D** shows the equivalent "CT angulation". The position of the pars marginalis is shown for comparison in D.

merely an oblique indentation in the lateral aspect of the second-trimester hemisphere. Over time it deepens and develops secondary sulci on the insular cortex, and the opercula portions of the surrounding frontal, parietal, and temporal lobes completely cover the insula, as described previously. The insular sulci form late. Garel did not see any evidence of the insular sulci before 31 weeks, and those structures were present in only 10% of 31-week fetuses. Insular sulci were present in all 36-week gestational age fetuses. Imaging of the fetal

brain in the axial plane allows good assessment of developing opercularization. The anterior and posterior lips of the opercula are everted up to 20 weeks' gestational age, but rapid cortical/subcortical growth causes the lips to grow toward each other, a process that is quite advanced by 26 weeks' gestational age. Garel assessed this development by measuring the distance between the anterior and posterior opercula and found few cases where the interopercular distance was less than 10 mm before 29 weeks. The distance then gradually reduced so that at 36 weeks' gestation, for example, 80% of values were between 4 and 8 mm. However, the opercula did not close completely before birth in any of the cases, so this event appears to occur postnatally. Cortical malformations may disrupt this process, but underopercularization without obvious structural abnormality is one of the "soft" neuroradiologic features seen with high frequency in children with developmental delay.

The central and precentral sulci are early features on the lateral surface of the developing hemispheres, with the central sulcus appearing first. Both structures are best assessed on axial imaging of the fetal brain. Garel found that the central sulcus was seen in 20% of her cases at 22 to 23 weeks, in 75% of cases at 26 weeks, and in all cases thereafter. Our experience is broadly comparable, although we saw the central sulcus consistently in 25- to 26-week fetuses on iuMR imaging. In contrast, the precentral sulcus was not shown by Garel before 26 weeks but was seen in 90% of 28-week fetuses and consistently after that time. The parieto-occipital sulcus is best appreciated on sagittal images of the fetus. It is visible after 22 weeks' gestational age in the vast majority of, if not all, fetuses.

OTHER SULCI OF IMPORTANCE FOR FETAL IMAGING

Superior and Inferior Frontal Sulci

Both of these sulci are best assessed on coronal images of the fetal brain. The data from Garel suggest the two sulci appear at approximately the same time, although fetuses with superior frontal sulci without inferior frontal gyri, but not vice versa, are a common finding. Both sulci are seen in a minority of fetuses at 26 weeks but in a majority at 27 weeks. Both sulci are consistently seen at 30 weeks and after.

Cingulate Sulcus

This sulcus was seen in two thirds of 22- to 23-week fetuses in Garel's cohort and was consistently visualized after that time. A similar schedule was demonstrated for the callosal sulcus, which is situated between the cingulate gyrus and the corpus callosum. Both of these sulci are best visualized on coronal iuMR images.

Superior and Inferior Temporal Sulci

Garel distinguished between the anterior and posterior portions of the superior temporal sulcus. We found that the anterior portion can be located with greater certainty, so we discuss the anterior portion of the superior temporal sulcus and the inferior temporal sulcus only. The coronal plane is required to assess both of these sulci, which appear to show much greater variation than the structures listed earlier. Neither is routinely seen before 27 weeks, but both are consistently seen after 33 weeks. Garel showed that more than 50%

of fetuses had definable superior temporal sulci by 31 weeks and inferior temporal sulci by 30 weeks.

Calcarine Sulcus

This feature of the medial portion of the occipital lobe is well-visualized on both coronal and sagittal images close to the midline. It is seen in two thirds of 22- to 23-week fetuses and in all fetuses after 25 weeks' gestation.

Collateral Sulcus

The coronal plane is optimal for assessing this sulcus, although ensuring that some of the rhinal sulcus is not included, particularly on 5-mm-thick sections, may be difficult. This sulcus is visualized in more than 50% of cases at 26 weeks and in all normal fetuses at 28 weeks and later.

The overall results of fetal sulcation are summarized in Table 1-1. Much more work is needed in this field in order to obtain more robust data. Garel's textbook did not extend back before 22 weeks' gestational age, and the number of cases under 25 weeks is limited. This is unfortunate because of the great need to understand normality in second-trimester fetuses so that robust interpretation of abnormal cases can be made. A corollary of this in clinical practice is the urgent need for research on the gestational age at which neocortical formation abnormalities can be confidently diagnosed or excluded. For example, lissencephaly is an uncommon malformation of cortical development, and the imaging features of lissencephaly are well described. Most cases show an absence or paucity of sulci with wide, abnormal gyri, which produce smooth hemispheric surfaces. If the only diagnostic feature of lissencephaly is lack of sulcation, how can the condition be diagnosed in the fetus when the normally developing

TABLE 1-1	
Summary of Fetal Sulcation Milestones	
Gestational Age (weeks)	**Sulcus Visualization**
22–24	100% visualization of • Median interhemispheric fissure • Lateral sulcus • Parieto-occipital sulcus • Calcarine sulcus • Cingulate sulcus
26	New sulci visible in the majority of cases • Central sulcus • Precentral sulcus • Collateral sulcus
30	New sulci visible in the majority of cases • Inferior temporal sulcus
31	New sulci visible in the majority of cases • Superior temporal sulcus (anterior portion)

Data from Garel C (ed): MRI of the Fetal Brain. Berlin, Springer-Verlag, 2004.

early brain is agyric? Although many cases of pediatric lissencephaly do have abnormal thickening of the cerebral cortex, this may not be obvious while the cortex is still developing in utero. The accuracy of in utero imaging in diagnosing lissencephaly at different stages of pregnancy is not known. In our experience, the vast majority of cases are not diagnosed by antenatal ultrasound in the second trimester, and it seems that iuMR also misses many cases of the subtler abnormalities of cortical formation in the second trimester. Therefore performing further studies of normal sulcation in the second-trimester fetus is vital because, for now, such

studies appear to be the only chance for early detection of abnormalities such as lissencephaly. This may be an overoptimistic view, however, remembering that pathologists have said for many years that accurate assessment of gestational age by inspection of fetal brains (certainly within 2 weeks) is not possible. The following figures show the normal changes in the surface appearance of the fetal brain between 19 and 37 weeks gestational age. Please note that there has been no attempt to scale the images with respect to the different gestational ages for purposes of anatomical clarity.

REFERENCES

1. Naidich TP, Brightbill TC: The pars marginalis I. A "bracket" sign for the central sulcus in axial plane CT and MRI. Int J Neuroradiol 2:3–19, 1996.
2. Naidich TP, Kang E, Fatterpekar G, et al: The insula: Anatomic study and MR imaging at 1.5 T. Am J Neuroradiol 25:222–232, 2004.
3. Feess-Higgins A, Larroche J-C (eds): Development of the Human Foetal Brain: An Anatomical Atlas. Paris, INSERM CNRS, 1987.
4. Stranding S (ed): Gray's Anatomy, 39th ed. Edinburgh, Elsevier, 2005.
5. Naidich TP, Valavanis AG, Kubik S: Anatomic relationships along the low-middle convexity: Part 1—Normal specimens and MR imaging. Neurosurgery 36:517–531, 1995.
6. Garel C (ed): MRI of the Fetal Brain. Berlin, Springer-Verlag, 2004.
7. Chi JG, Dooling EC, Gilles FH: Gyral development of the human brain. Ann Neurol 1:86–93, 1977.

SUPERIOR SURFACE

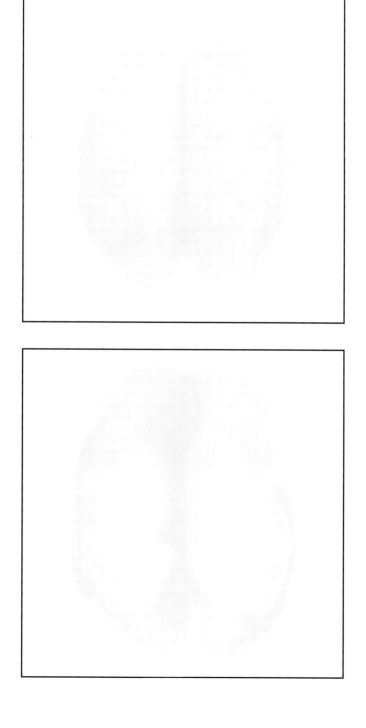

Median longitudinal fissure

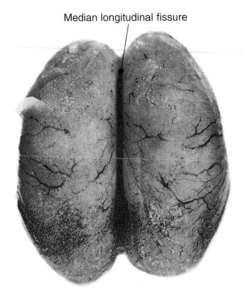

SUPERIOR SURFACE, 19–20 WEEKS

Median longitudinal fissure

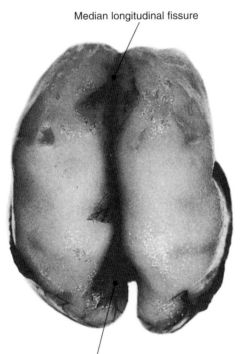

SUPERIOR SURFACE, 22–23 WEEKS   Parieto-occipital sulcus

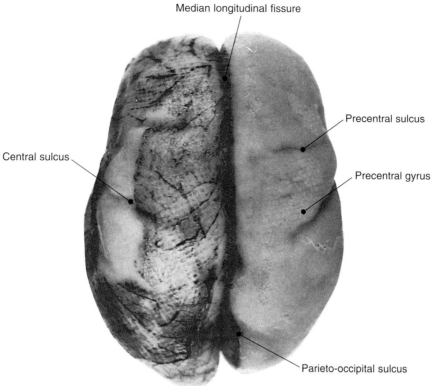

Median longitudinal fissure

Precentral sulcus

Precentral gyrus

Central sulcus

Parieto-occipital sulcus

SUPERIOR SURFACE, 25–26 WEEKS

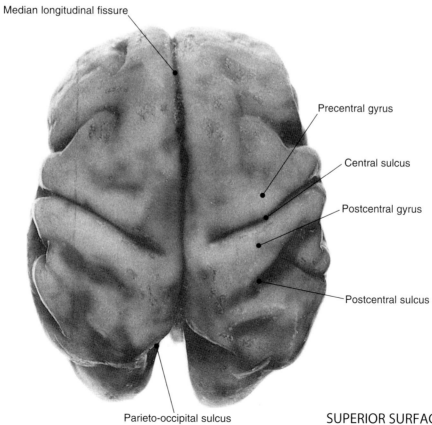

Median longitudinal fissure

Precentral gyrus

Central sulcus

Postcentral gyrus

Postcentral sulcus

Parieto-occipital sulcus

SUPERIOR SURFACE, 28–29 WEEKS

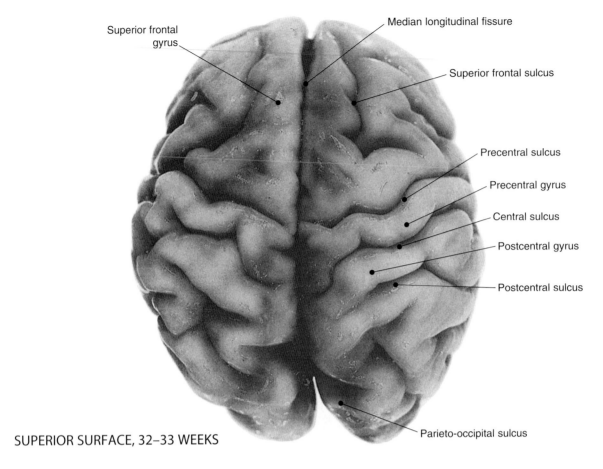

Superior frontal gyrus

Median longitudinal fissure

Superior frontal sulcus

Precentral sulcus

Precentral gyrus

Central sulcus

Postcentral gyrus

Postcentral sulcus

Parieto-occipital sulcus

SUPERIOR SURFACE, 32–33 WEEKS

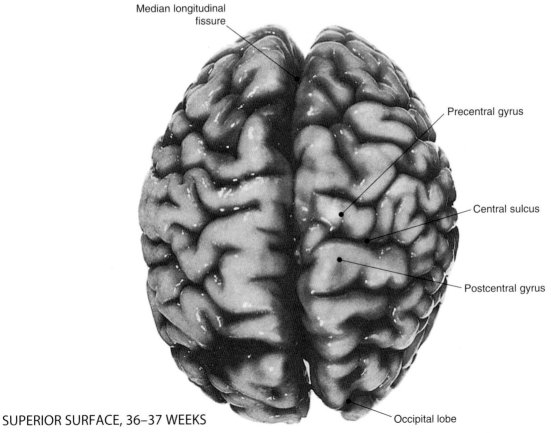

Median longitudinal fissure

Precentral gyrus

Central sulcus

Postcentral gyrus

Occipital lobe

SUPERIOR SURFACE, 36–37 WEEKS

LATERAL SURFACE

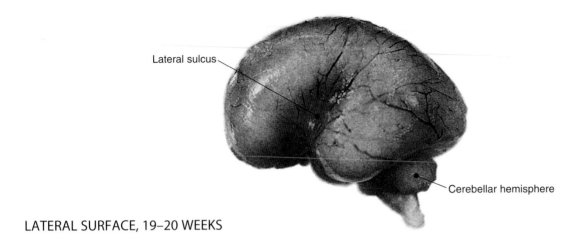

Lateral sulcus

Cerebellar hemisphere

LATERAL SURFACE, 19–20 WEEKS

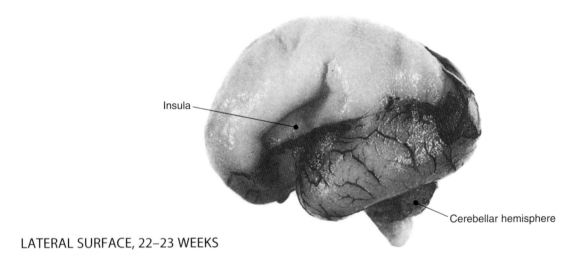

Insula

Cerebellar hemisphere

LATERAL SURFACE, 22–23 WEEKS

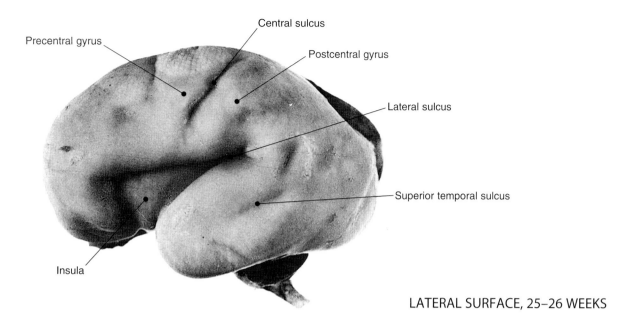

Precentral gyrus

Central sulcus

Postcentral gyrus

Lateral sulcus

Superior temporal sulcus

Insula

LATERAL SURFACE, 25–26 WEEKS

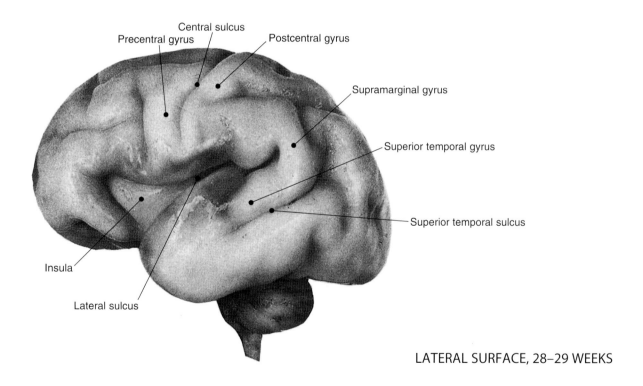

Central sulcus

Precentral gyrus

Postcentral gyrus

Supramarginal gyrus

Superior temporal gyrus

Superior temporal sulcus

Insula

Lateral sulcus

LATERAL SURFACE, 28–29 WEEKS

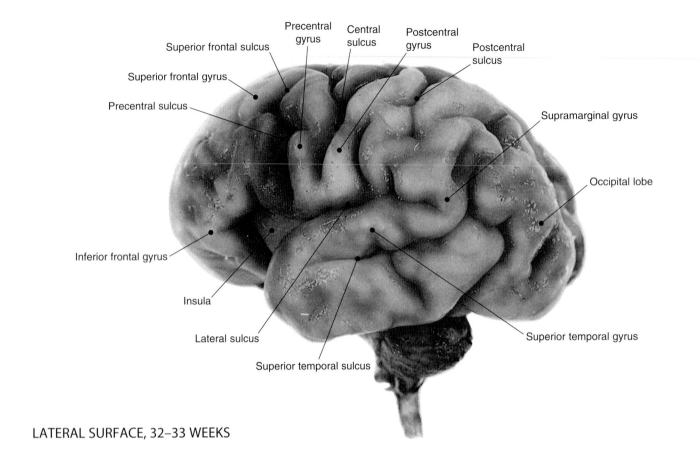

LATERAL SURFACE, 32–33 WEEKS

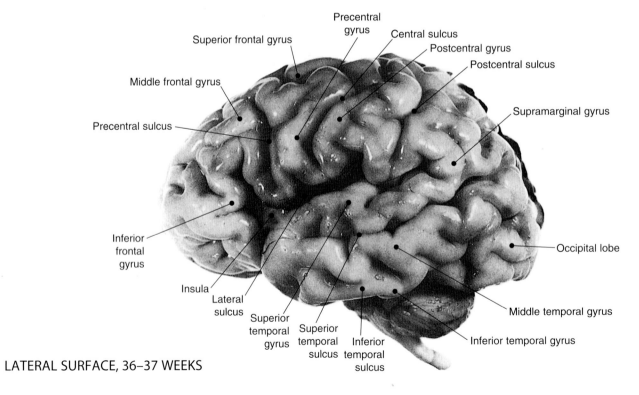

LATERAL SURFACE, 36–37 WEEKS

INFERIOR SURFACE

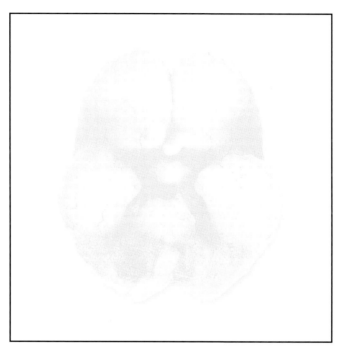

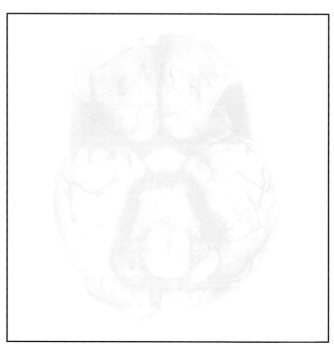

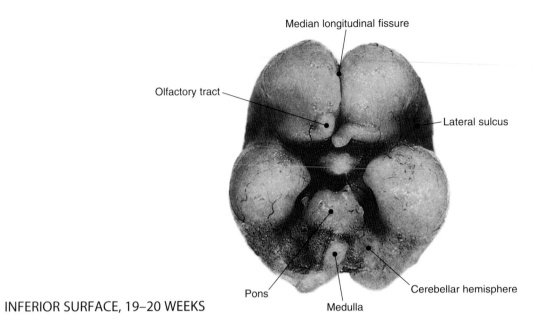

Median longitudinal fissure

Olfactory tract

Lateral sulcus

Pons

Medulla

Cerebellar hemisphere

INFERIOR SURFACE, 19–20 WEEKS

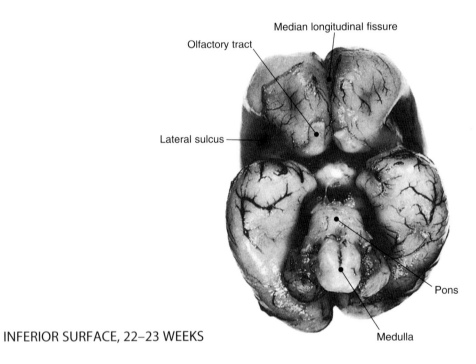

Median longitudinal fissure

Olfactory tract

Lateral sulcus

Pons

Medulla

INFERIOR SURFACE, 22–23 WEEKS

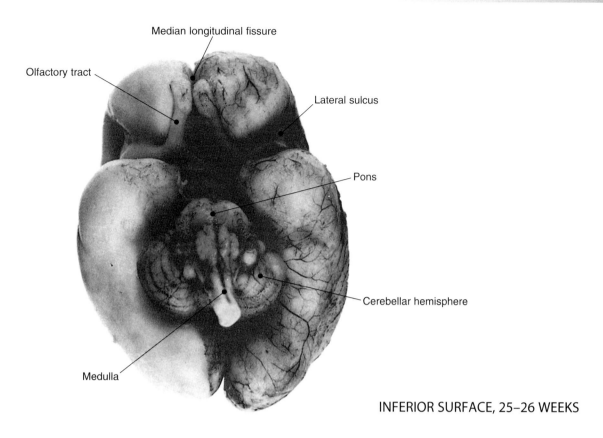

Median longitudinal fissure

Olfactory tract

Lateral sulcus

Pons

Cerebellar hemisphere

Medulla

INFERIOR SURFACE, 25–26 WEEKS

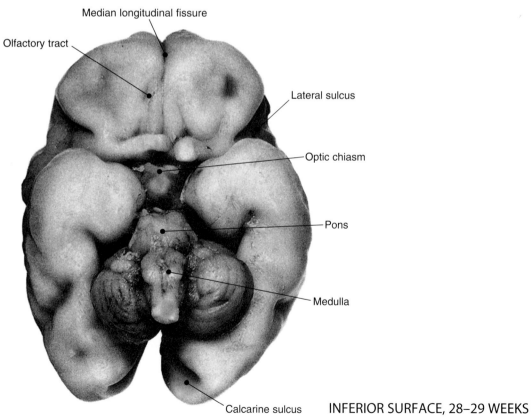

Median longitudinal fissure

Olfactory tract

Lateral sulcus

Optic chiasm

Pons

Medulla

Calcarine sulcus

INFERIOR SURFACE, 28–29 WEEKS

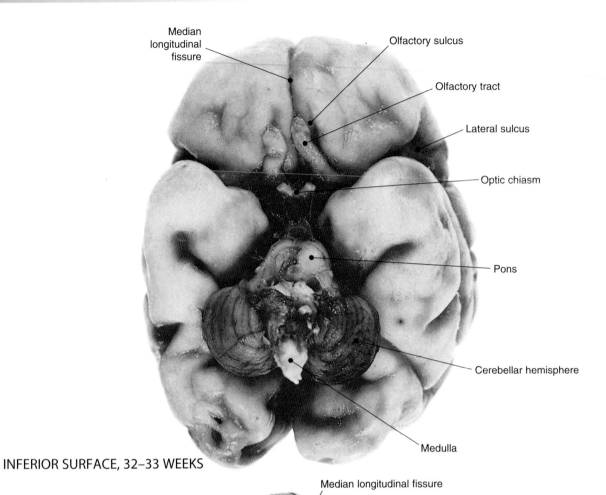

Median longitudinal fissure

Olfactory sulcus

Olfactory tract

Lateral sulcus

Optic chiasm

Pons

Cerebellar hemisphere

Medulla

INFERIOR SURFACE, 32–33 WEEKS

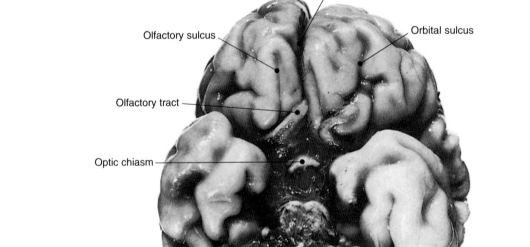

Median longitudinal fissure

Olfactory sulcus

Orbital sulcus

Olfactory tract

Optic chiasm

Cerebellar hemisphere

INFERIOR SURFACE, 36–37 WEEKS

MEDIAL SURFACE

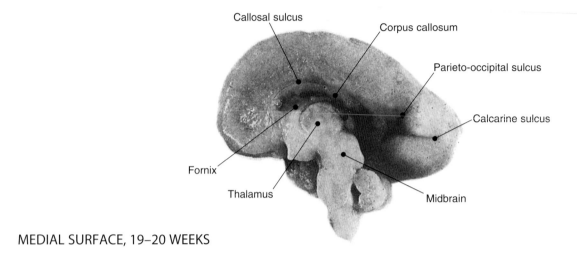

MEDIAL SURFACE, 19–20 WEEKS

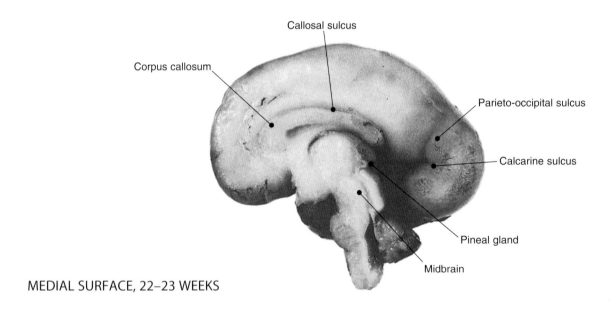

MEDIAL SURFACE, 22–23 WEEKS

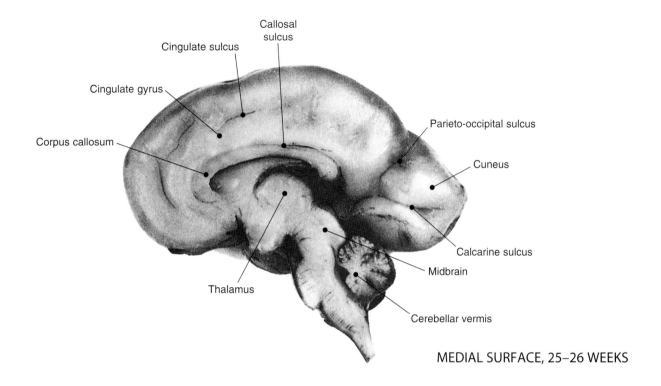

Callosal sulcus

Cingulate sulcus

Cingulate gyrus

Parieto-occipital sulcus

Corpus callosum

Cuneus

Calcarine sulcus

Midbrain

Thalamus

Cerebellar vermis

MEDIAL SURFACE, 25–26 WEEKS

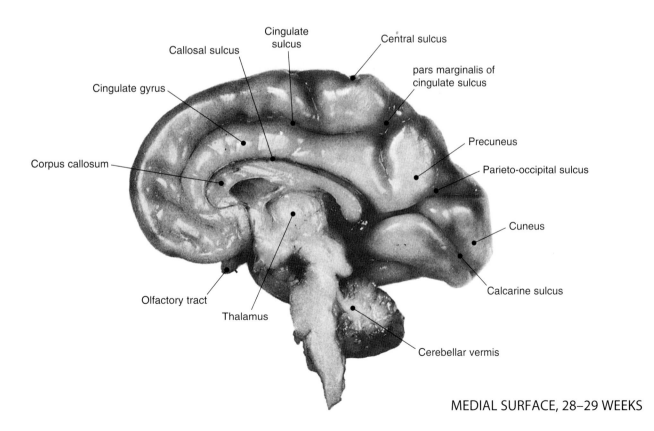

Cingulate sulcus

Central sulcus

Callosal sulcus

pars marginalis of cingulate sulcus

Cingulate gyrus

Precuneus

Corpus callosum

Parieto-occipital sulcus

Cuneus

Calcarine sulcus

Olfactory tract

Thalamus

Cerebellar vermis

MEDIAL SURFACE, 28–29 WEEKS

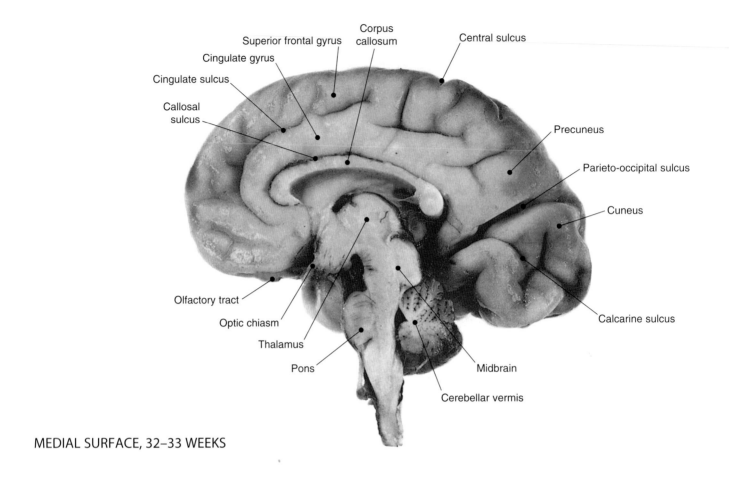

MEDIAL SURFACE, 32–33 WEEKS

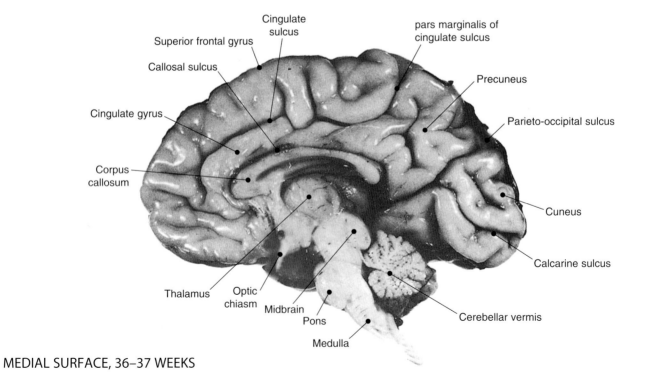

MEDIAL SURFACE, 36–37 WEEKS

SECTIONAL ANATOMY OF THE FETAL BRAIN

The major part of this section is a pictorial review of cross-sectional fetal brain anatomy using magnetic resonance (MR) imaging matched as closely as possible with postmortem histologic sections. It should be appreciated that by the time the fetal brain has reached 19 to 20 weeks (the earliest fetal images shown in this text), all of the major structural components visible in routine neuroradiologic practice have formed and are clearly visible. Because of this, previous knowledge of adult neuroanatomy can be used to a large extent; indeed, the basic neuroanatomy does not change during this period. The difficulty in interpreting fetal and neonatal imaging arises in the evolving anatomic features of the brain. We discussed the evolution of the "sulcated brain" at the start of Section 1 and myelination is discussed in Section 3, which covers postnatal imaging. The purpose of this section is to give an introduction to the transient structures in the wall of the developing fetal brain, that is, structures that are not found in the adult, pediatric, or even the term newborn brain.

TRANSIENT STRUCTURES IN THE FETAL CEREBRAL HEMISPHERES

The original Larroche atlas used anatomic terminology from the *Nomina Anatomica* of the International Anatomical Nomenclature Committee.[1] As explained in the introduction of the Larroche atlas, some anatomic features are not fully covered by *Nomina Anatomica*, particularly structures peculiar to the developing brain. The authors made reference to more specific papers, such as the work of Rakic and Yakovlev[2] and Angevine et al.[3] in order to assist with nomenclature. The two main structures that are found in the fetus but not in the brain of adults or children are the subependymal germinative zones ("germinal matrix") and the transient laminated structures found in the developing cerebral hemispheres. The latter arise from the ventricofugal migration of neurons and glia toward the future cortex and deep gray matter structures. Recently, there has been considerable interest and research in the development of the cerebral cortex in the human fetus. The second trimester is an exceptionally active period of neuronal/glial cell birth, proliferation, and migration. MR imaging has played a role because it allows visualization of the normal structures of the developing cerebral hemispheres, which appear to correspond to the features shown on histologic studies.[4] This has had important clinical repercussions for classifying neocortical brain malformations on pediatric neuroimaging.[5,6]

One of the striking macroscopic and histologic features of the fetal brain is the presence of large germinal matrices adjacent to the ventricles, which are particularly prominent in the second-trimester fetus.[7] The primary germinal matrix or neuroepithelium is a cell-dense structure that lines the cerebral ventricles. Those cells proliferate extensively and produce neurons, glia, and the secondary germinal matrix. Bayer and Altman[7] found that the secondary germinal matrix (or subventricular zone) produces mainly neurons that are destined to become cortical interneurons and astrocytes. Some of the secondary germinal matrices migrate away from the ventricles and complete their cell-producing role at sites distant from the ventricles. Leading among these are the matrices that form the granule, basket and stellate cells of the cerebellar cortex, and granule cells in the dentate gyrus of the hippocampus.

At some sites in the brain of the second-trimester fetus the germinal matrix is particularly large and is named by the structures that ultimately will be produced. For example, large neuroepithelial/subventricular zones are found around the lateral ventricles and are called the *striatal matrices* because they will form the putamen and caudate. Feess-Higgins and Larroche used terms such as *matrix rhombencephalica*, *matrix mesencephalica*, and *matrix telencephalica* in their atlas (but labeled simply as *matrix* in the figures of the original text) to distinguish the anatomic site of the germinal matrix and therefore imply the structures formed from those regions of neural/glial proliferation. In this atlas we simply use the term *germinal matrix* in our annotation in the hope that which portion of the ventricular system is adjacent is obvious. This simplification does not undervalue the importance of the germinal matrix from either a developmental or an imaging point of view. On the contrary, the germinal matrix is a prominent landmark on fetal MR imaging, particularly in the second trimester, and may hold the key to early detection of some disorders of cortical formation.

The germinal matrix is one of the few structures in the normal fetal brain that has very short T2 values (i.e., appears dark on T2-weighted images). This feature provides superb contrast between the high signal of the cerebrospinal fluid in the ventricles on its deep surface and the intermediate signal of the developing brain superficially. This tissue contrast is exceptionally well seen on postmortem MR (pmMR) because of the lack of time constraints that allow the use of sequences with low echo train lengths and high number of excitations. The contrast resolution of the germinal matrix is sometimes poor on in utero MR (iuMR) using single-shot fast spin echo (SSFSE) sequences. This is partly due to the low sensitivity to susceptibility changes because of the blurring brought about as a result of the high number of echoes in the sequence (T2 decay k-space filtering). The primary and secondary germinal matrices can be shown and differentiated on histologic studies. On MR imaging, however, the two structures cannot be resolved even on high-resolution pmMR because they are so closely opposed and have identical signal characteristics. The pmMR images in this atlas show the primary and secondary matrices clearly on 19- to 20-week, 22- to 23-week, and 25- to 26-week fetuses, and the matrices can often be seen on iuMR at these gestational ages. However, by 29 to 30 weeks, the germinal matrices are less distinct on pmMR, and by 32 to 33 weeks they can be seen only in a minority of sites.

The other transient structures that are of great interest to researchers in the field are the laminar, cellular compartments within the developing cerebral wall that ultimately will govern the organized formation of the cortex and other subcortical gray matter regions of the cerebral hemispheres. Bayer and Altman[7] discuss the historical approach to describing the developing cerebral mantle and explain the new developments in understanding the process. The classic description of the second-trimester cerebral cortex involves only three layers: the deep, periventricular germinal matrix that forms the neurons and glia, the superficial cortical plate (which will become layers 2–6 of the neocortex), and an intermediate zone. The intermediate zone recently has come under particular scrutiny by some groups. Its microscopic anatomy reveals a highly complex, regionally specific pattern called "stratified transitional fields" by Altman and Bayer[7,8] and the "transient fetal zones" by Kostovic et al.[9,10] One component of the intermediate zone is the huge number of radial glial cells extending through the full thickness of the hemisphere. Further-more, Kostovic et al showed that those glial structures guide the migration of cells formed in the germinal matrix to a predetermined site in the developing cortex by a process called *fate mapping*. Those radial fibers cannot be resolved on MR imaging, although their presence can be inferred in some developmental abnormalities such as focal cortical dysplasias and cortical tubers associated with tuberous sclerosis complex.[11] The observations by Bayer and Altman stress, however, that the intermediate zone should not be viewed as a passive structure, merely allowing the transit of neurons and glia *en passant*. Instead it is an important region where cell migration is arrested to allow stratification and early synaptic contact. The authors suggest that "precortical" interactions are vital for normal cortical development. By implication the intermediate zone must be an important area of further imaging research in cases where the neocortex does not form properly.

Bland and Altman describe six different regions in the intermediate zone: stratified transitional fields 1 to 6 (i.e., STF1 [superficial] through to STF6 [abutting the germinal matrix]). These strata develop in the first trimester but undergo considerable growth in the second trimester and for the most part have undergone involution in the third trimester, although some portions persist to become the established mature white matter. Histologically, significant differences between the STF strata in regions will become "sensory regions," with large numbers of granular cells in layer IV (granular cortex) in the mature brain, and the "motor regions" with greater numbers of pyramidal cells in layer V (agranular cortex). In principle, knowledge of the strata and their contents can help explain the regional differences in MR signal seen in the second-trimester fetal brain on pmMR and, to a lesser extent, on iuMR.

STF1 lies just below the cortical plate and is a relatively thick structure. It contains mainly fibrous structures with a large proportion of free extra-cellular fluid and few cell bodies. It has high signal on T2-weighted images in contrast to the low-signal cortical plate superficially. It is seen in both granular and agranular cortices and will become the subcortical white matter. STF2 and STF3 are cell-rich regions and are the last "sojourn" site before neurons and glia enter the cortical plate. STF2 is most prominent in agranular cortex; STF3 is found only in granular cortical regions. Both of these structures have disappeared in the mature brain. STF4, STF5, and STF6 are fibrous, cellular, and fibrous, respectively. STF5 is thought to be the first "sojourn" site of migrating cells; STF4 will become the deep white matter; and the last-to-form STF6 contributes primarily to callosal fibers. These structures are seen well on histologic studies, and STF2 to STF6 can be clearly delineated from STF1 superficially and the deeper germinal matrix on pmMR. Areas of regional heterogeneity within STF2 to STF6 are seen on pmMR, but how they relate to the histologically defined regions has not yet been determined.

It would be of great value if the wealth of information from histologic studies on human fetuses could be used to improve our understanding and interpretation of fetal

TABLE 2-1		
Overview of Stages of Development of the Cerebral Cortex and White Matter		
	Gestational Age (Converted to Post Last Menstrual Period)	**Main Features**
Embryonic	Phase I: 6–9 weeks	Universal embryonic zone
Early fetal	Phase II: 10–14 weeks	Formation of cortical plate
Mid fetal	Phase III: 15–17 weeks	Formation of transient fetal zones
	Phase IV: 18–26 weeks	Peak of subplate zone
Late fetal	Phase V: 27–38 weeks	Dissolution of transient fetal zones
Neonate	Phase VI	Immature six-layer cortex

Modified from Rados M, Judas M, Kostvic I: In vitro MRI of brain development. Eur J Radiol 57:187–198, 2006.

imaging studies. Interpretation of MR images without direct comparison with histologic studies is fraught with problems; fortunately, Rados et al.[4] have made significant inroads into the subject. Many of the details described here are seen well on pmMR images, particularly on the coronal sections of 19- to 20-week and 22- to 23-week fetuses. Rados et al. used a different nomenclature system for the transient layers in the wall of the cerebral hemispheres of the second- and third-trimester fetus than did Bayer and Altman, what might be considered a more "classic" system. They studied fetuses from all three trimesters, and their overall view of the development of the cerebral cortex is summarized in Table 2-1.

Rados et al. describe the early fetal brain (10–13 weeks postovulatory weeks, therefore approximately 12–15 weeks post last menstrual period) as having the standard three-layer structure, namely, cortical plate, intermediate zone, and ventricular zone. By the midfetal period (which they defined as 15–22 weeks postovulatory weeks, approximately 17–24 weeks post last menstrual period) the transient zones have developed, and the authors describe seven layers demonstrable on histologic studies. From superficial to deep they are as follows (Figure 2-1):

1. Marginal zone: Not visible in neocortical regions on pmMR studies
2. Cortical plate
3. Subplate zone
4. Intermediate zone
5. Subventricular zone
6. Fiber-rich periventricular zone
7. Ventricular zone: Equivalent to the primary and secondary germinal matrices of Bayer and Altman

Rados et al. place great importance on the subplate zone in the normal development of the cerebral cortex; it reaches its developmental peak at 27 to 30 weeks postovulatory weeks (approximately 29–32 weeks post last menstrual period). They note that the subplate is the largest single component of the cerebral wall in the second-trimester fetus and that it is proportionally much larger in human fetuses than in fetuses of other mammalian species. Although the subplate does contain cell bodies of both neurons and glia, Rados et al. consider the subplate to be the major "waiting" compartment for fibers that are destined to project to the future

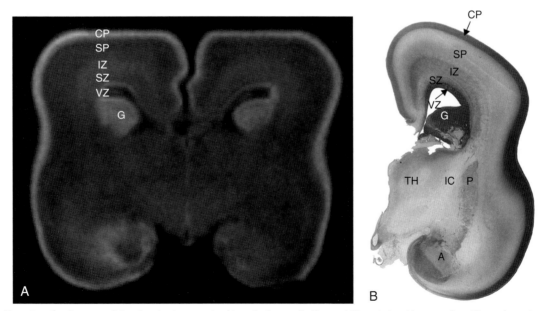

Figure 2-1   Transient fetal zones of the developing cerebral hemispheres. **A,** Coronal T1-weighted image of an 18-week postovulatory week fixed fetal brain (20 weeks post last menstrual period). **B,** Histologic section from a 20- to 21-week postovulatory week fixed fetal brain (22–23 weeks post last menstrual period). *CP,* Cortical plate; *IC,* internal capsule; *IZ,* intermediate zone; *G,* germinal matrix; *P,* putamen *SP,* subplate, *SZ,* subventricular zone; *TH,* thalamus; *VZ,* ventricular zone. (From Rados M, Judas M, Kostvic I: In vitro MRI of brain development. Eur J Radiol 57:187–198, 2006.)

mature cerebral cortex. They detailed the major axonal contributors to the subplate in earlier publications[9], which include thalamocortical projections, projections from the basal forebrain, and ipsilateral and cortico–cortical projections via the corpus callosum. It is suspected that modeling and parcellation of the future cerebral cortex is instigated at this time.

The subplate zone also appears to have a significant effect on the morphologic development of the sulcal/gyral pattern of the future cerebral cortex. Kostovic cites the following supporting evidence:

- The subplate zone is much thinner in species that have smooth oligogyric brains in mature animals.
- Within the human brain, there is greater gyration in the regions that have the thickest subplate zone.
- The frontal lobes continue to develop tertiary gyri postnatally, and this is accompanied by persistence of the subplate zone in those regions.

Rados et al. used their extensive experience in fetal histology to explain the signal characteristics of the transient fetal layers on MR imaging. It should be appreciated that major differences exist between their methods of pmMR and those we present in this atlas. They performed pmMR on brains that had been fixed with aldehyde after removal from the body, whereas we used pmMR on unfixed tissue with the fetal brain still in situ. In those circumstances, they found that T1-weighted images were best for second-trimester fetuses, whereas T2-weighted images gave better results in more mature fetuses. In contrast, we used T2-weighted sequences throughout the gestational age ranges studied. In spite of this, similar interpretation of the signal characteristics likely is valid for our studies as well. The two regions of the second-trimester fetal cerebral hemisphere that have the highest cellular density are the ventricular zone (germinal matrix) and the cortical plate. Those regions returned high signal on the T1-weighted pmMR studies of Rados et al. and low signal on our T2-weighted pmMR studies. This is not surprising because we know from other imaging studies that regions that have high cellular density and high nuclear-to-cytoplasmic ratios (e.g., primitive neuroectodermal tumors and lymphoma) have T1 and T2 shortening in comparison to normal brain. In contrast, the subplate zone has a high proportion of extracellular components that are intensely hydrophilic. Therefore the high water content in the subplate zone is responsible for the low signal on T1-weighted images and the high signal on T2-weighted images. This is true at least in fetuses at 30 weeks' gestation post last menstrual period, but from then on the disappearance of the extracellular, hydrophilic matrix produces blurring between the subplate and intermediate zone (and to a lesser extent between the subplate and cortical plate).

The appearance of the other transient layers of the second-trimester fetus (intermediate zone, fiber-rich periventricular zone, and subventricular zone) is more difficult to resolve on MR. This is because of the reduced inherent contrast resolution between the adjacent layers and intense regional and temporal variations. Judging by the images of the second-trimester fetus shown in the Rados paper, T1-weighted images of fixed tissue appear to discriminate between those structures better than T2-weighted images of unfixed tissue. However, the basic principles appear to hold true: regions with high cellularity (e.g., cortical plate) have comparatively high signal on T1-weighted images and low signal on T2-weighted images, whereas the reverse signal pattern is seen in cell-sparse regions (subplate zone). These features are summarized in Table 2-2.

The reasons why the rapid SSFSE T2-weighted sequences used for in utero fetal imaging discriminate between germinal matrix and fetal brain with less clarity than do short echo train length FSE T2-weighted sequences used for pmMR have already been discussed. Those arguments also hold true for the transient fetal structures of the developing cerebral hemisphere. That is not to say that they cannot be seen in utero, because in some cases they can, but in our experience not in a robust fashion. The development of the germinal matrix and transient hemispheric structures must hold the key to the abnormal development of many cortical malformations, and this warrants further research and development of imaging methods to show those structures with greater clarity. This is not a problem in fetuses postmortem, and interesting features can be shown in developmental abnormalities. An example is shown in Figure 2-2.

Some improvements have been made in delineating the transient zones of the fetus using iuMR, particularly with refinements of diffusion-weighted imaging (DWI). This is a difficult sequence to use in utero but has been shown to be possible by many groups. Most frequently DWI is performed with an echoplanar imaging method using its "ultrafast" capability. The signal contrast produced on DWI and the associated apparent diffusion coefficient (ADC) map is dependent on how freely water can diffuse on a microscopic scale. In regions where water diffusion is restricted, DWI shows very high signal matched by low-signal (low-diffusion) regions on the ADC maps (Figure 2-3). It is possible that further refinement of such techniques will contribute to improved early detection of subtle abnormalities of neocortical development.

TABLE 2-2

Summary of Signal Characteristics of Different Regions of the Developing Cerebral Hemispheric Wall of the Fetus on Magnetic Resonance Imaging

Zone	Predominant Histology	T1W Signal	T2W Signal
Cortical plate	Cell dense	↑	↓
Subplate	Extracellular hydrophilic matrix	↓	↑
Intermediate	Cellular	↑	↓
Subventricular	Cell sparse	↓	↑
Ventricular	Cellular	↑	↓

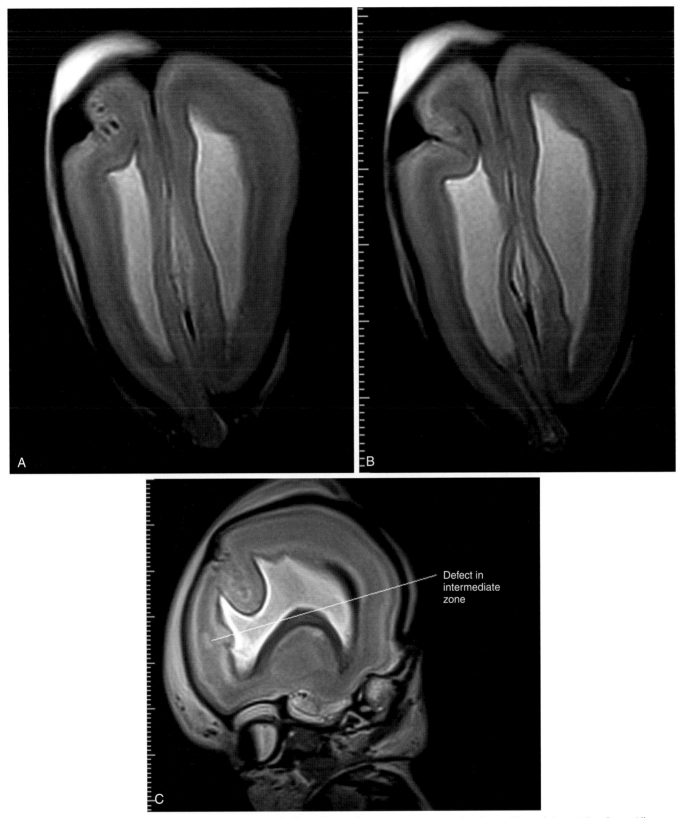

Defect in
intermediate
zone

Figure 2-2   Postmortem magnetic resonance imaging of a fetus that underwent spontaneous abortion at 19 weeks' gestational age. All images are T2-weighted. **A, B,** Images in the axial plane at the level of the superior portions of the ventricles. Both hemispheres are abnormal, showing ventriculomegaly, but the right hemisphere also has a parietal meningoencephalocystocele and an abnormal cleft with an anomalous venous structure in it adjacent to the right frontal lobe. Note that the intermediate zone is markedly thinner in the right hemisphere which is shown well on parasagittal imaging **(C)** along with a focal defect as indicated.

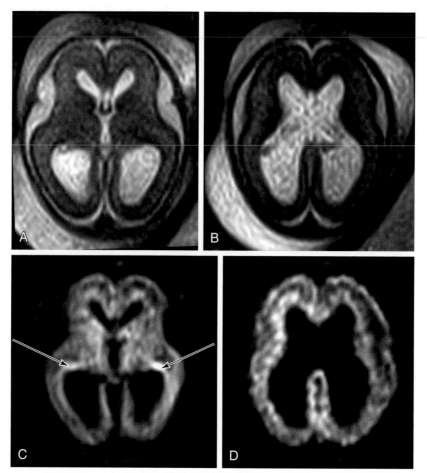

Figure 2-3   Examples of diffusion-weighted imaging in a 22-week fetus with isolated ventriculomegaly. **A, B,** Single-shot fast spin echo images in the axial plane through the ventricles. **C, D,** Equivalent diffusion-weighted images (b = 1000). Note that the germinal matrix has high signal on diffusion-weighted images *(arrows)* indicating low diffusivity, and the subplate has low signal on diffusion-weighted imaging indicating high diffusivity.

REFERENCES

1. International Anatomical Nomenclature Committee: Nomina Anatomica, 5th ed. Baltimore, Williams & Wilkins, 1983.
2. Rakic P, Yakovlev PI: Development of the corpus callosum and cavum septi in man. J Comp Neurol 132:45–72, 1968.
3. Angevine JB, Mancall EL, Yakovlev PI: The Human Cerebellum. An Atlas of Gross Topography in Serial Sections. Boston, Little Brown & Co., 1961.
4. Rados M, Judas M, Kostovic I: In vitro MRI of brain development. Eur J Radiol 57:187–198, 2006.
5. Dobyns WB, Truwit CL: Lissencephaly and other malformations of cortical development: 1995 update. Neuropediatrics 26:132–147, 1995.
6. Barkovich AJ, Kuzniecky RI, Dobyns WB, et al: A classification scheme for malformations of cortical development. Neuropediatrics 27:59–63, 1996.
7. Bayer SA, Altman J: Atlas of Human CNS Development: Volume 3—The Human Brain During the Second Trimester. Boca Raton, FL, CRC Press, 2005.
8. Altman J, Bayer SA: Regional differences in the stratified transitional field and the honeycomb matrix of the developing human cerebral cortex. J Neurocytol 31:613–632, 2002.
9. Kostovic I, Rakic P: Developmental history of the transient subplate zone in the visual and somatosensory cortex of the macaque monkey and human brain. J Comp Neurol 297:441–470, 1990.
10. Kostovic I, Judas M, Rados M, Hrabac P: Laminar organization of the human fetal cerebrum revealed by histochemical markers and MR imaging. Cereb Cortex 12:536–544, 2002.
11. Griffiths PD, Bolton P, Verity C: White matter abnormalities in tuberous sclerosis complex. Acta Radiol 39:482–486, 1998.

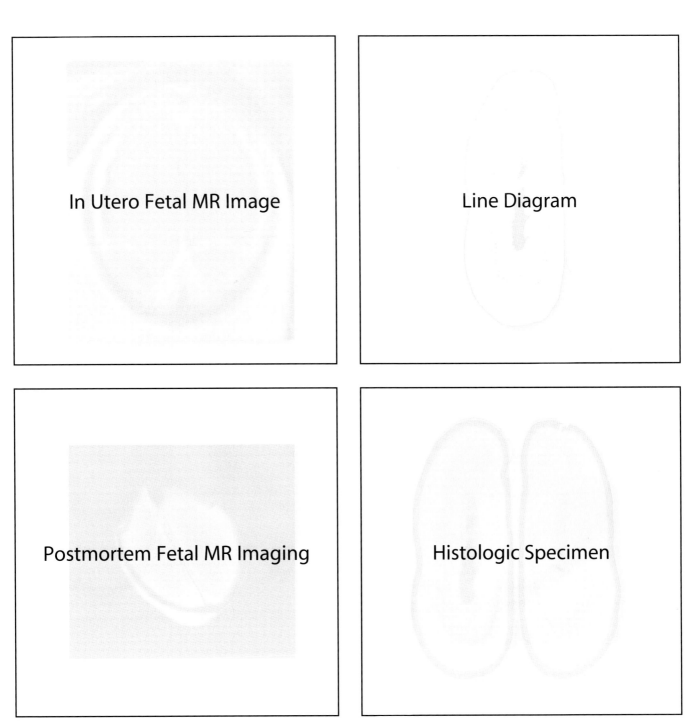

In Utero Fetal MR Image

Line Diagram

Postmortem Fetal MR Imaging

Histologic Specimen

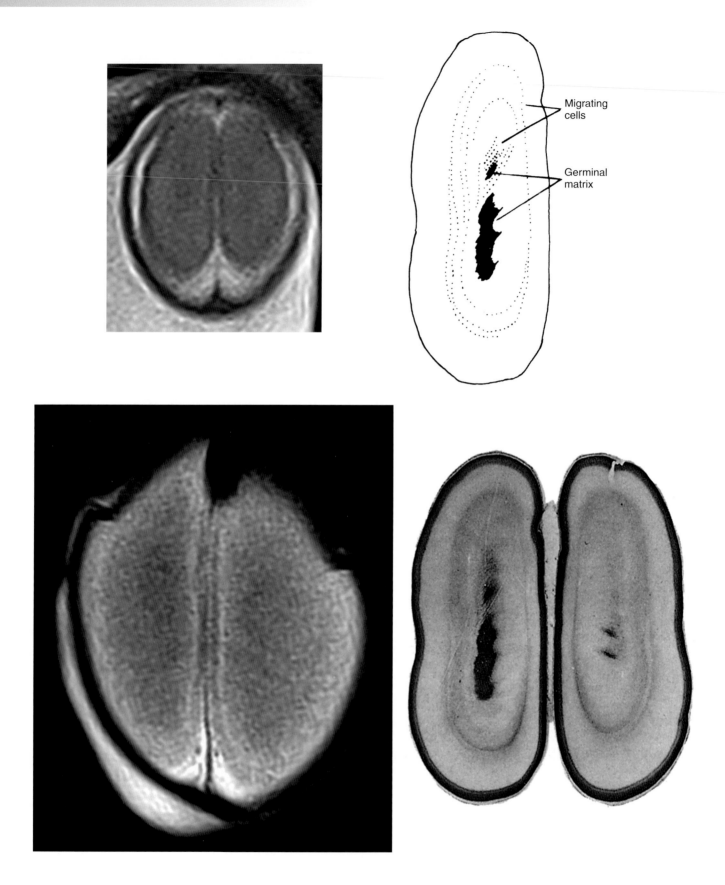

Migrating cells

Germinal matrix

19–20 WEEKS GESTATIONAL AGE, AXIAL SECTION

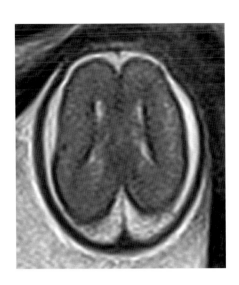

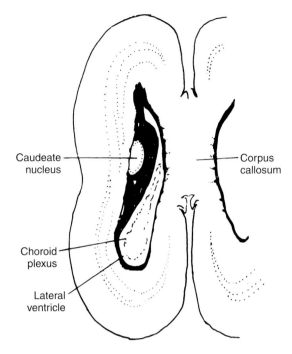

Caudeate nucleus

Corpus callosum

Choroid plexus

Lateral ventricle

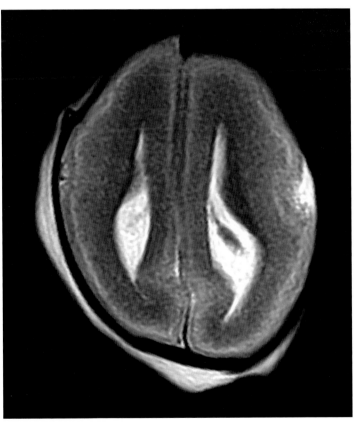

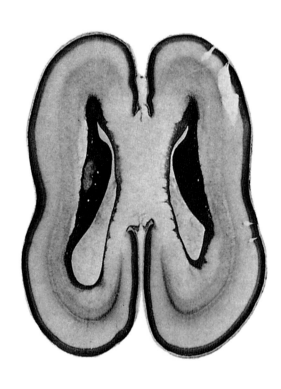

19–20 WEEKS GESTATIONAL AGE, AXIAL SECTION

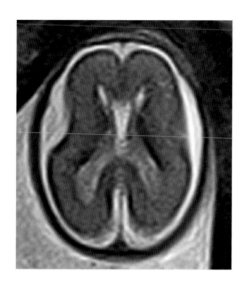

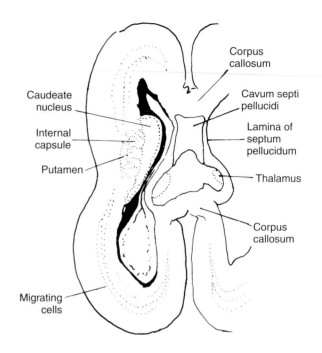

Caudeate nucleus

Internal capsule

Putamen

Migrating cells

Corpus callosum

Cavum septi pellucidi

Lamina of septum pellucidum

Thalamus

Corpus callosum

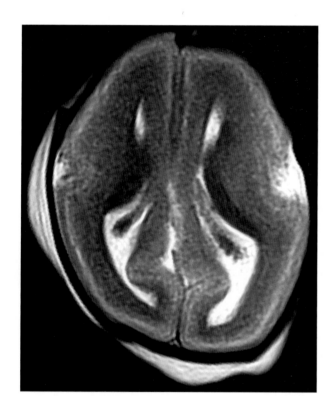

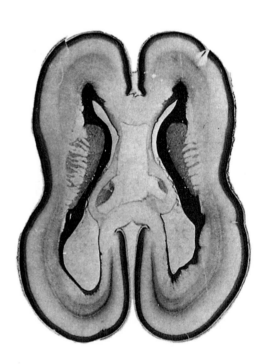

19–20 WEEKS GESTATIONAL AGE, AXIAL SECTION

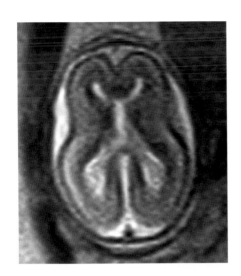

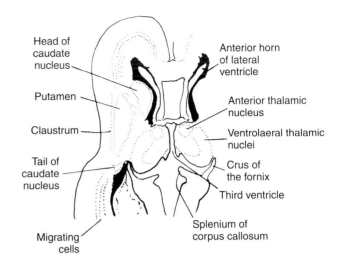

Head of
caudate
nucleus

Putamen

Claustrum

Tail of
caudate
nucleus

Migrating
cells

Anterior horn
of lateral
ventricle

Anterior thalamic
nucleus

Ventrolaeral thalamic
nuclei

Crus of
the fornix

Third ventricle

Splenium of
corpus callosum

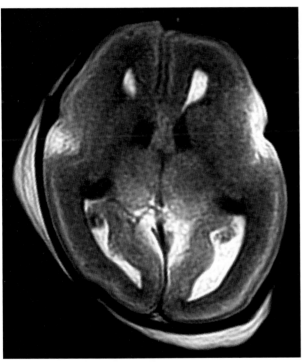

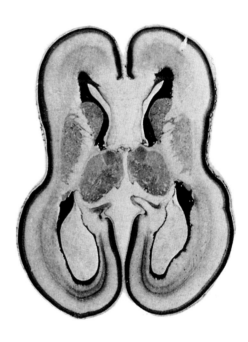

19–20 WEEKS GESTATIONAL AGE, AXIAL SECTION

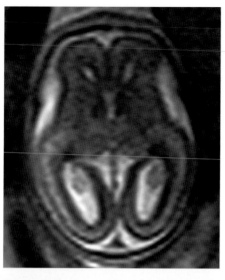

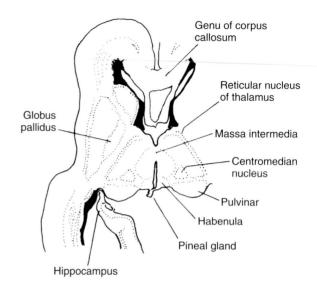

Genu of corpus callosum

Reticular nucleus of thalamus

Globus pallidus

Massa intermedia

Centromedian nucleus

Pulvinar

Habenula

Pineal gland

Hippocampus

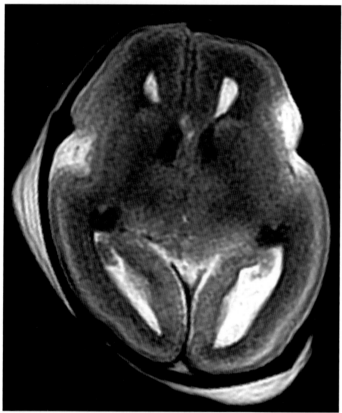

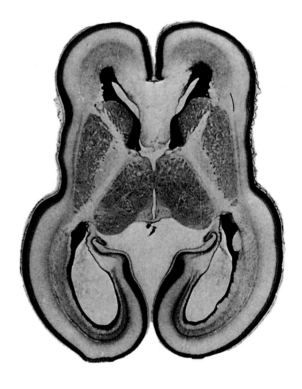

19–20 WEEKS GESTATIONAL AGE, AXIAL SECTION

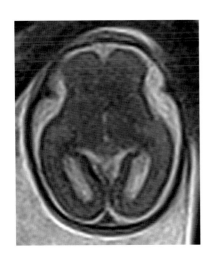

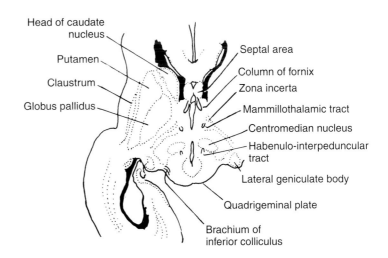

Head of caudate nucleus

Putamen

Claustrum

Globus pallidus

Septal area

Column of fornix

Zona incerta

Mammillothalamic tract

Centromedian nucleus

Habenulo-interpeduncular tract

Lateral geniculate body

Quadrigeminal plate

Brachium of inferior colliculus

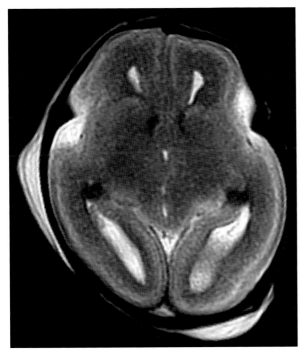

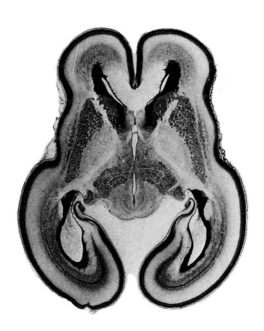

19–20 WEEKS GESTATIONAL AGE, AXIAL SECTION

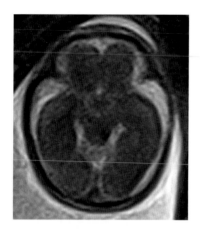

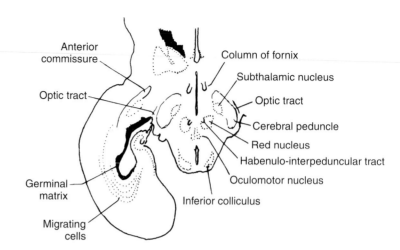

Anterior commissure

Optic tract

Germinal matrix

Migrating cells

Column of fornix

Subthalamic nucleus

Optic tract

Cerebral peduncle

Red nucleus

Habenulo-interpeduncular tract

Oculomotor nucleus

Inferior colliculus

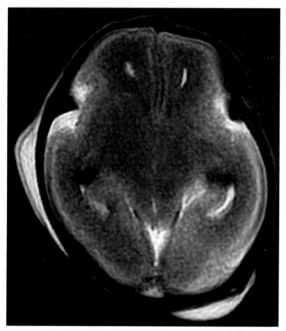

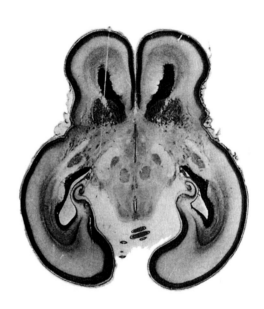

19–20 WEEKS GESTATIONAL AGE, AXIAL SECTION

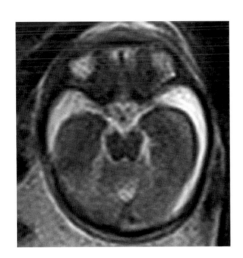

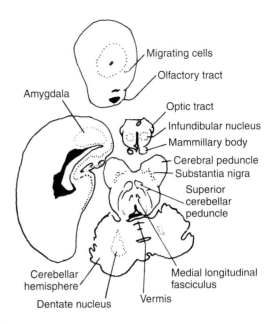

Migrating cells

Olfactory tract

Amygdala

Optic tract

Infundibular nucleus

Mammillary body

Cerebral peduncle

Substantia nigra

Superior
cerebellar
peduncle

Cerebellar
hemisphere

Medial longitudinal
fasciculus

Dentate nucleus

Vermis

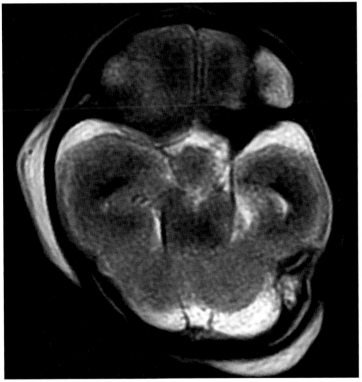

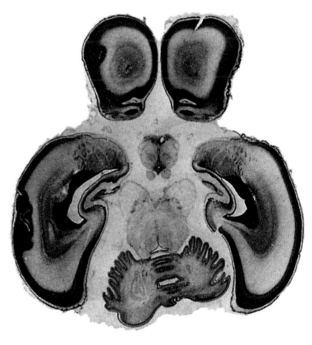

19–20 WEEKS GESTATIONAL AGE, AXIAL SECTION

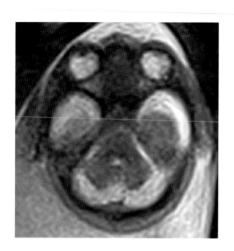

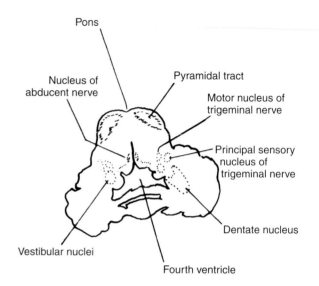

Pons

Nucleus of
abducent nerve

Pyramidal tract

Motor nucleus of
trigeminal nerve

Principal sensory
nucleus of
trigeminal nerve

Dentate nucleus

Vestibular nuclei

Fourth ventricle

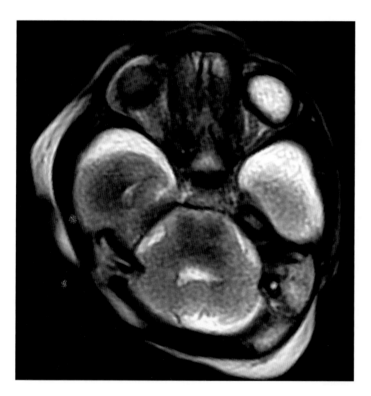

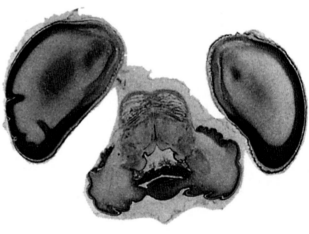

19–20 WEEKS GESTATIONAL AGE, AXIAL SECTION

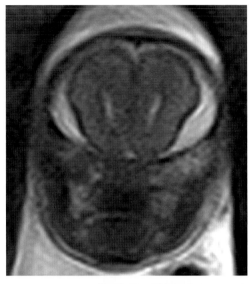

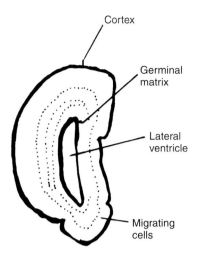

Cortex

Germinal matrix

Lateral ventricle

Migrating cells

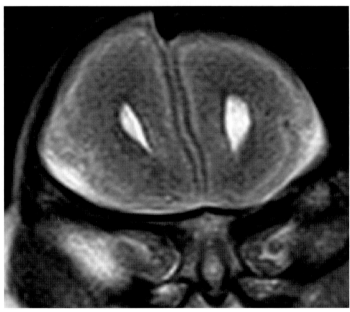

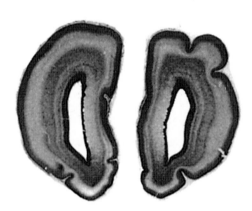

19–20 WEEKS GESTATIONAL AGE, CORONAL SECTION

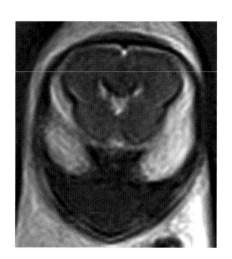

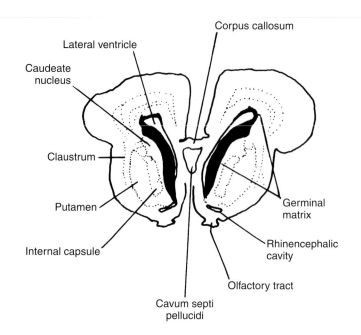

Caudeate
nucleus

Lateral ventricle

Corpus callosum

Claustrum

Putamen

Internal capsule

Cavum septi
pellucidi

Olfactory tract

Rhinencephalic
cavity

Germinal
matrix

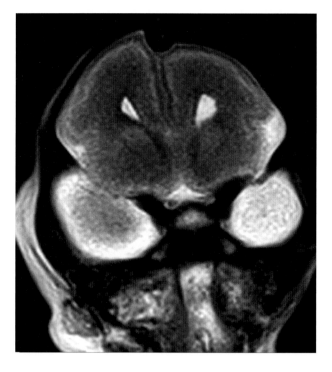

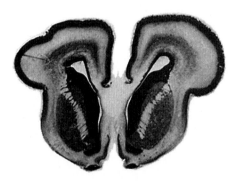

19–20 WEEKS GESTATIONAL AGE, CORONAL SECTION

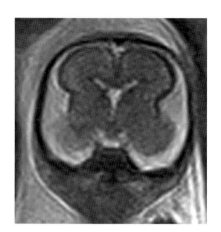

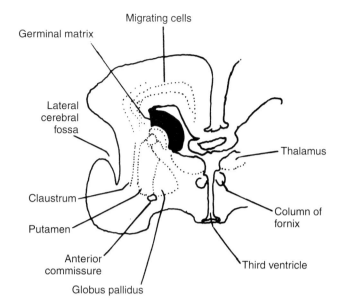

Migrating cells

Germinal matrix

Lateral
cerebral
fossa

Thalamus

Claustrum

Column of
fornix

Putamen

Anterior
commissure

Third ventricle

Globus pallidus

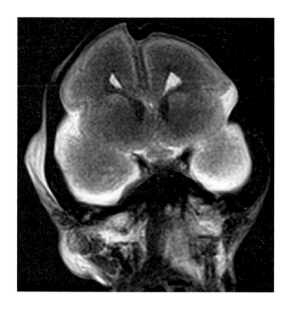

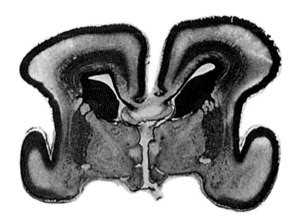

19–20 WEEKS GESTATIONAL AGE, CORONAL SECTION

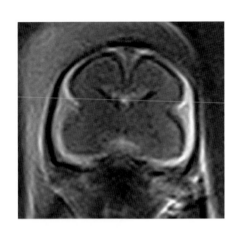

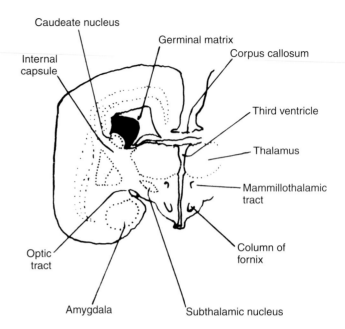

Caudeate nucleus

Germinal matrix

Corpus callosum

Internal capsule

Third ventricle

Thalamus

Mammillothalamic tract

Optic tract

Column of fornix

Amygdala

Subthalamic nucleus

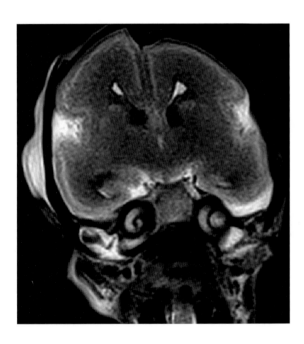

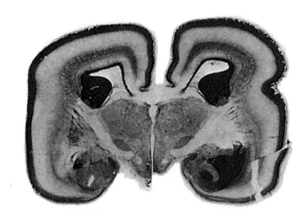

19–20 WEEKS GESTATIONAL AGE, CORONAL SECTION

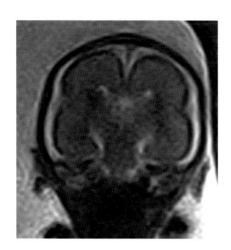

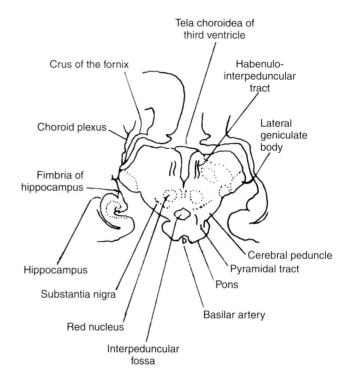

Tela choroidea of
third ventricle

Crus of the fornix

Habenulo-
interpeduncular
tract

Choroid plexus

Lateral
geniculate
body

Fimbria of
hippocampus

Cerebral peduncle

Hippocampus

Pyramidal tract

Substantia nigra

Pons

Red nucleus

Basilar artery

Interpeduncular
fossa

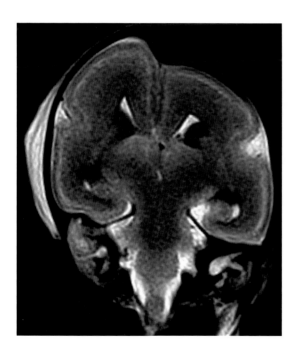

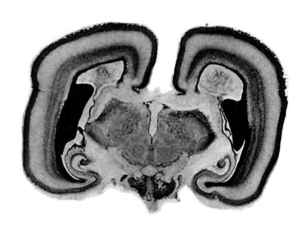

19–20 WEEKS GESTATIONAL AGE, CORONAL SECTION

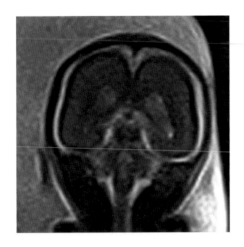

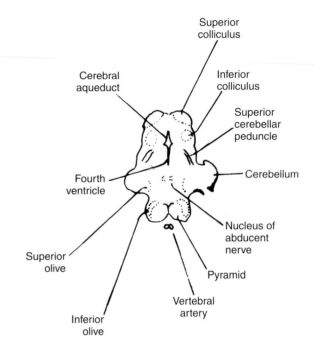

Superior colliculus

Cerebral aqueduct

Inferior colliculus

Superior cerebellar peduncle

Cerebellum

Fourth ventricle

Nucleus of abducent nerve

Superior olive

Pyramid

Vertebral artery

Inferior olive

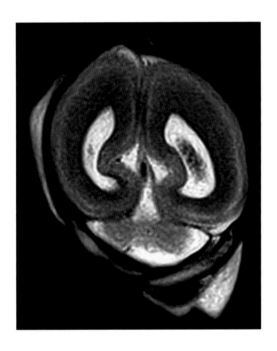

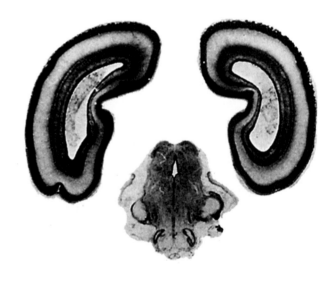

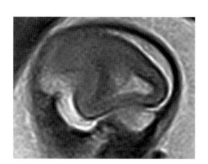

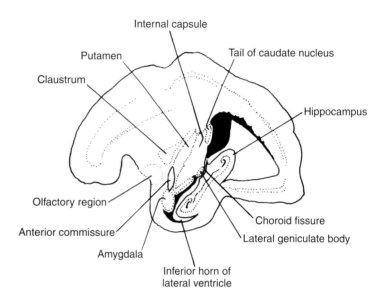

Internal capsule

Putamen

Claustrum

Tail of caudate nucleus

Hippocampus

Olfactory region

Anterior commissure

Amygdala

Inferior horn of
lateral ventricle

Choroid fissure

Lateral geniculate body

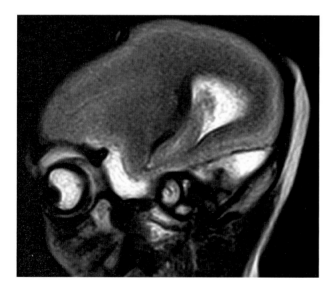

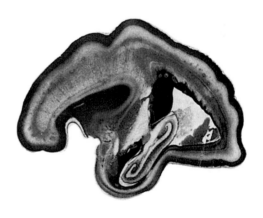

19–20 WEEKS GESTATIONAL AGE, SAGITTAL SECTION

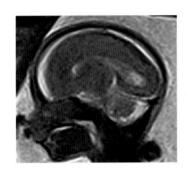

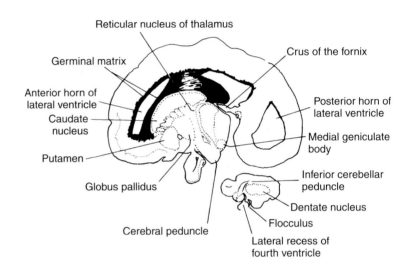

Reticular nucleus of thalamus

Germinal matrix

Crus of the fornix

Anterior horn of
lateral ventricle

Caudate
nucleus

Posterior horn of
lateral ventricle

Medial geniculate
body

Putamen

Globus pallidus

Inferior cerebellar
peduncle

Dentate nucleus

Flocculus

Cerebral peduncle

Lateral recess of
fourth ventricle

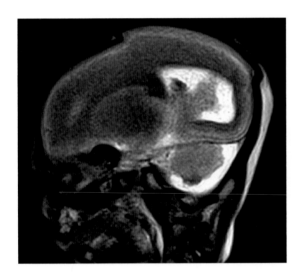

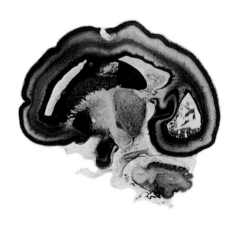

19–20 WEEKS GESTATIONAL AGE, SAGITTAL SECTION

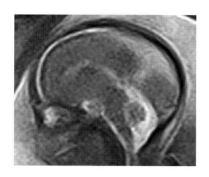

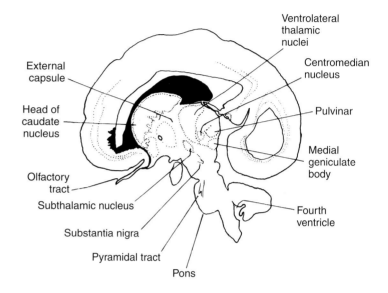

Ventrolateral
thalamic
nuclei

External
capsule

Centromedian
nucleus

Head of
caudate
nucleus

Pulvinar

Olfactory
tract

Medial
geniculate
body

Subthalamic nucleus

Fourth
ventricle

Substantia nigra

Pyramidal tract

Pons

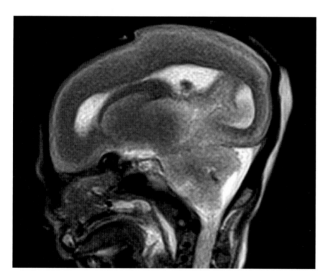

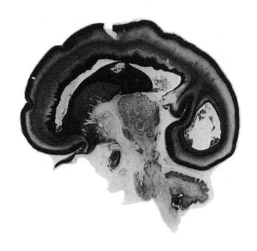

19–20 WEEKS GESTATIONAL AGE, SAGITTAL SECTION

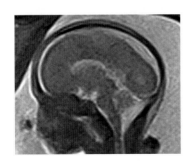

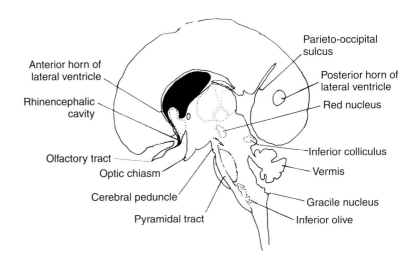

Anterior horn of lateral ventricle

Rhinencephalic cavity

Olfactory tract

Optic chiasm

Cerebral peduncle

Pyramidal tract

Parieto-occipital sulcus

Posterior horn of lateral ventricle

Red nucleus

Inferior colliculus

Vermis

Gracile nucleus

Inferior olive

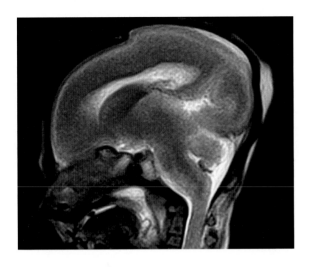

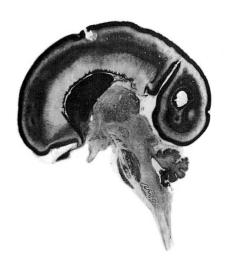

19–20 WEEKS GESTATIONAL AGE, SAGITTAL SECTION

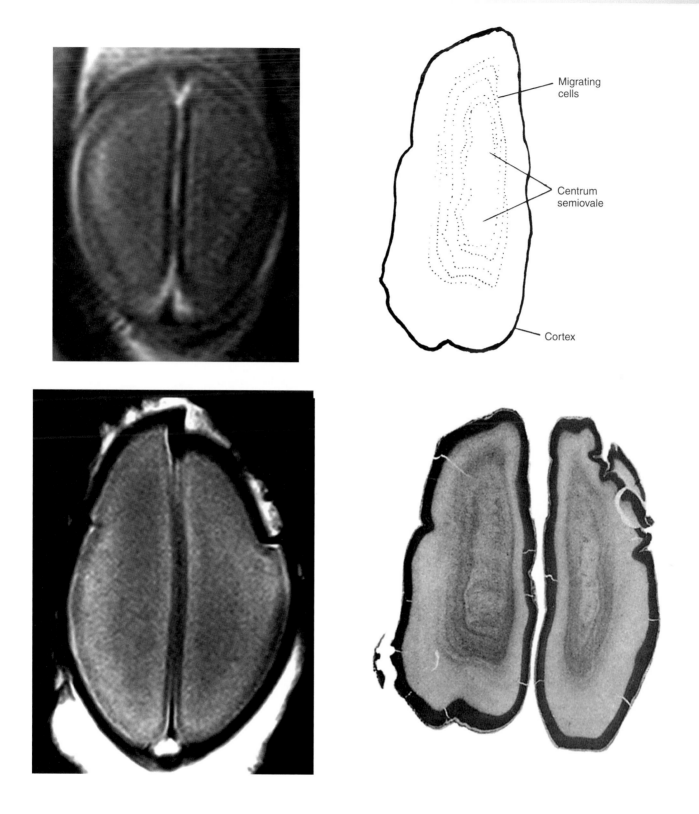

22–23 WEEKS GESTATIONAL AGE, AXIAL SECTION

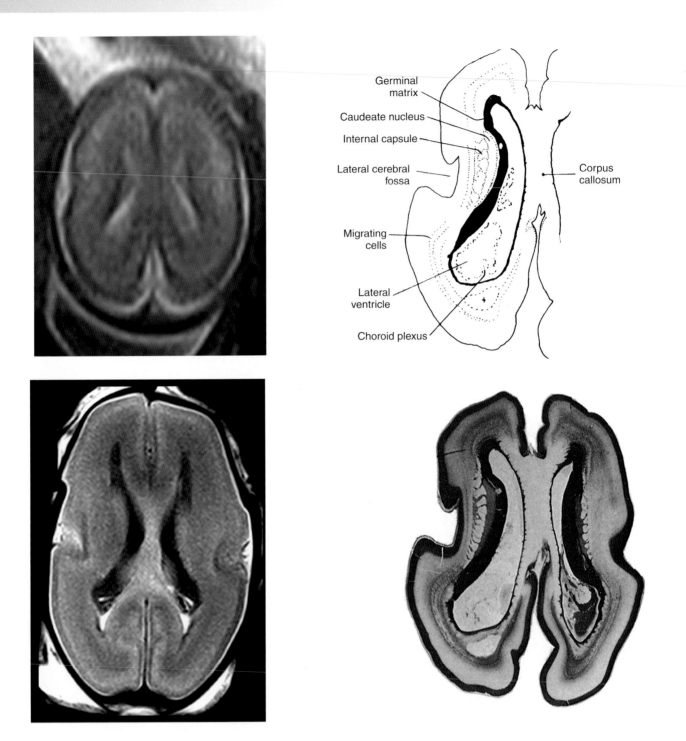

Germinal matrix

Caudeate nucleus

Internal capsule

Lateral cerebral fossa

Migrating cells

Lateral ventricle

Choroid plexus

Corpus callosum

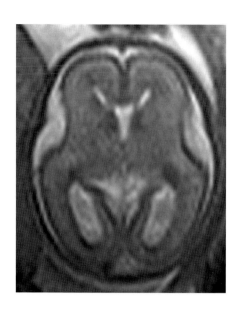

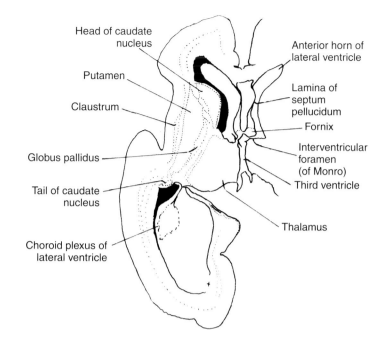

Head of caudate nucleus

Putamen

Claustrum

Globus pallidus

Tail of caudate nucleus

Choroid plexus of lateral ventricle

Anterior horn of lateral ventricle

Lamina of septum pellucidum

Fornix

Interventricular foramen (of Monro)

Third ventricle

Thalamus

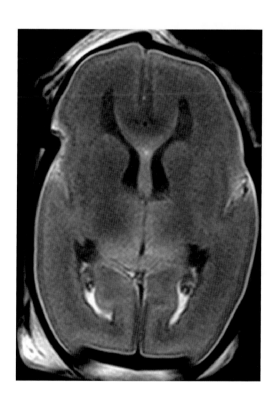

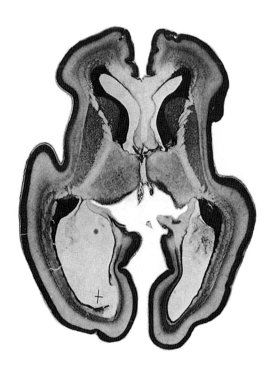

22–23 WEEKS GESTATIONAL AGE, AXIAL SECTION

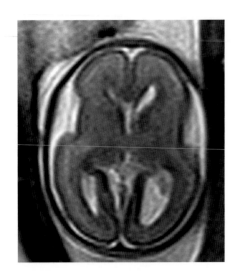

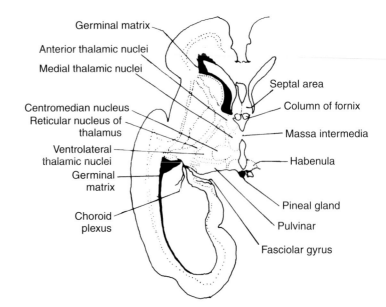

Germinal matrix

Anterior thalamic nuclei

Medial thalamic nuclei

Centromedian nucleus
Reticular nucleus of
thalamus
Ventrolateral
thalamic nuclei
Germinal
matrix

Choroid
plexus

Septal area

Column of fornix

Massa intermedia

Habenula

Pineal gland

Pulvinar

Fasciolar gyrus

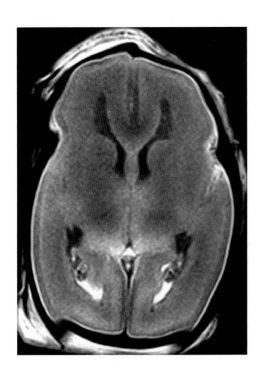

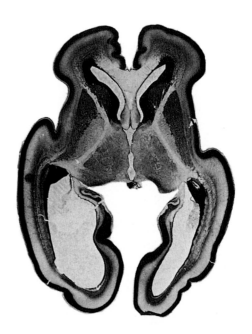

22–23 WEEKS GESTATIONAL AGE, AXIAL SECTION

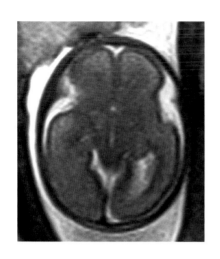

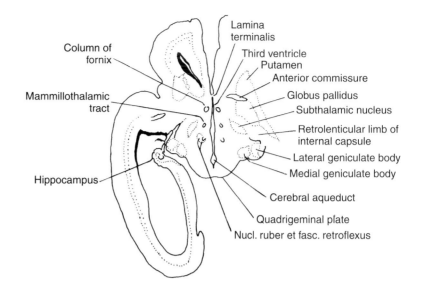

Column of fornix

Lamina terminalis

Third ventricle

Putamen

Anterior commissure

Globus pallidus

Subthalamic nucleus

Retrolenticular limb of internal capsule

Lateral geniculate body

Medial geniculate body

Cerebral aqueduct

Quadrigeminal plate

Nucl. ruber et fasc. retroflexus

Mammillothalamic tract

Hippocampus

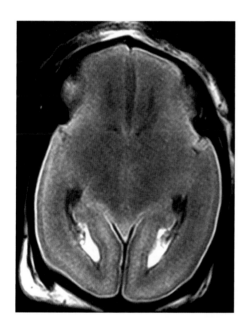

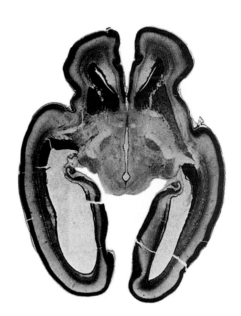

22–23 WEEKS GESTATIONAL AGE, AXIAL SECTION

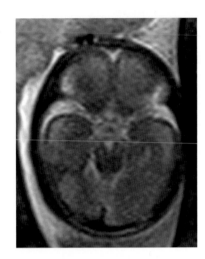

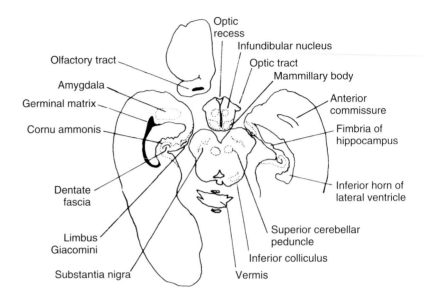

Optic recess
Infundibular nucleus
Olfactory tract
Optic tract
Amygdala
Mammillary body
Germinal matrix
Anterior commissure
Cornu ammonis
Fimbria of hippocampus
Dentate fascia
Inferior horn of lateral ventricle
Limbus Giacomini
Superior cerebellar peduncle
Inferior colliculus
Substantia nigra
Vermis

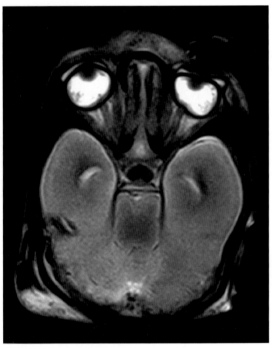

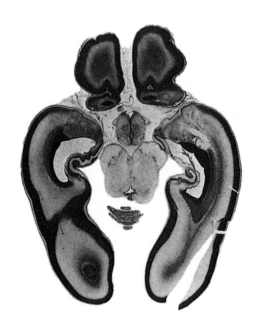

22–23 WEEKS GESTATIONAL AGE, AXIAL SECTION

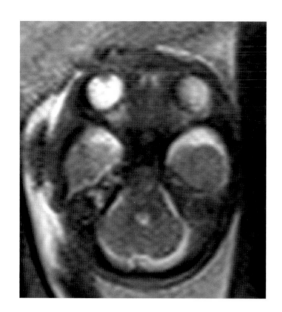

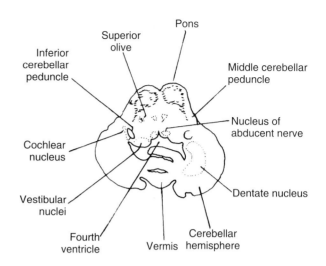

Superior olive

Pons

Inferior cerebellar peduncle

Middle cerebellar peduncle

Nucleus of abducent nerve

Cochlear nucleus

Vestibular nuclei

Fourth ventricle

Vermis

Cerebellar hemisphere

Dentate nucleus

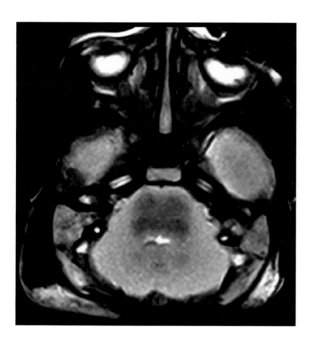

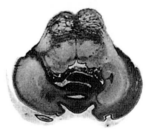

22–23 WEEKS GESTATIONAL AGE, AXIAL SECTION

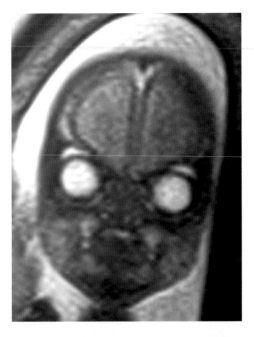

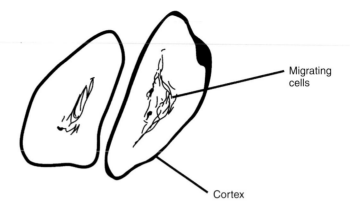

Migrating
cells

Cortex

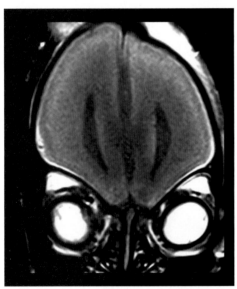

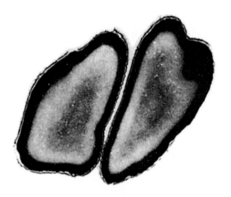

22–23 WEEKS GESTATIONAL AGE, CORONAL SECTION

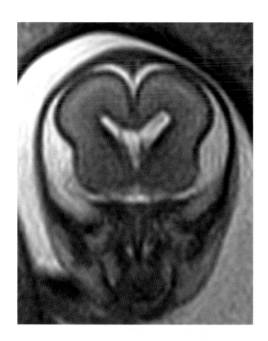

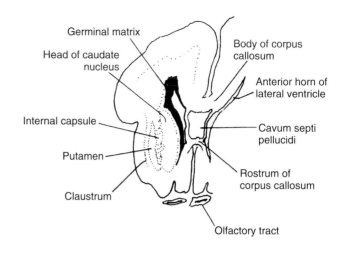

Germinal matrix

Head of caudate
nucleus

Body of corpus
callosum

Anterior horn of
lateral ventricle

Internal capsule

Cavum septi
pellucidi

Putamen

Rostrum of
corpus callosum

Claustrum

Olfactory tract

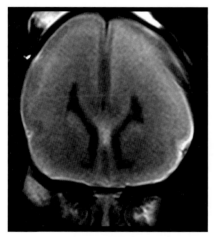

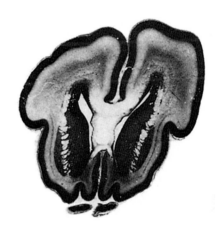

22–23 WEEKS GESTATIONAL AGE, CORONAL SECTION

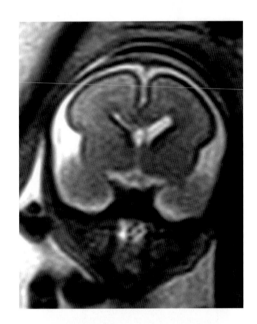

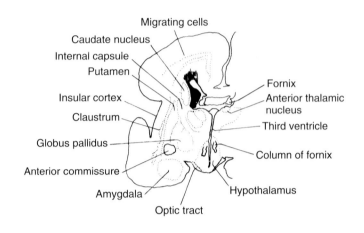

Migrating cells

Caudate nucleus
Internal capsule
Putamen

Fornix
Anterior thalamic
nucleus

Insular cortex

Third ventricle

Claustrum

Globus pallidus

Column of fornix

Anterior commissure

Hypothalamus

Amygdala

Optic tract

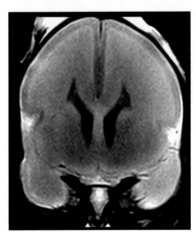

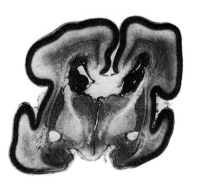

22–23 WEEKS GESTATIONAL AGE, CORONAL SECTION

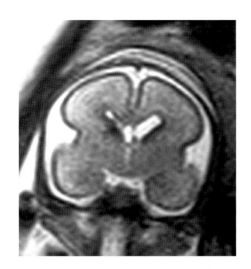

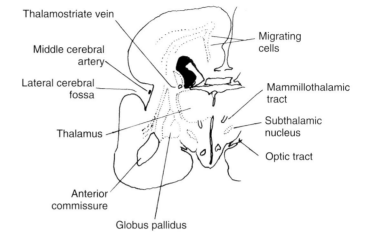

Thalamostriate vein

Middle cerebral
artery

Lateral cerebral
fossa

Thalamus

Anterior
commissure

Globus pallidus

Migrating
cells

Mammillothalamic
tract

Subthalamic
nucleus

Optic tract

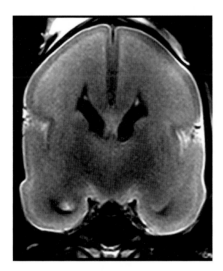

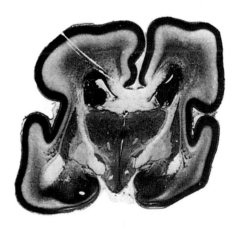

22–23 WEEKS GESTATIONAL AGE, CORONAL SECTION

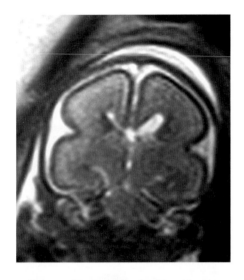

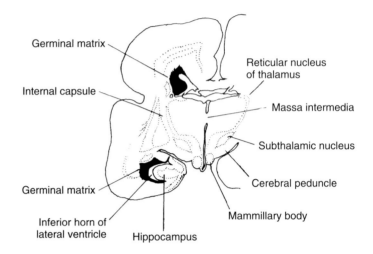

Germinal matrix

Reticular nucleus
of thalamus

Internal capsule

Massa intermedia

Subthalamic nucleus

Cerebral peduncle

Germinal matrix

Mammillary body

Inferior horn of
lateral ventricle

Hippocampus

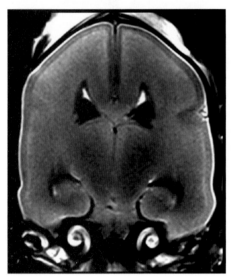

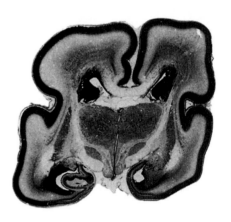

22–23 WEEKS GESTATIONAL AGE, CORONAL SECTION

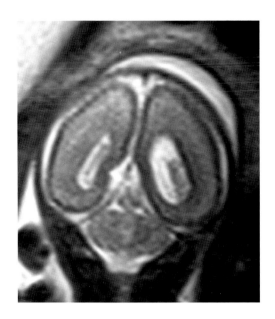

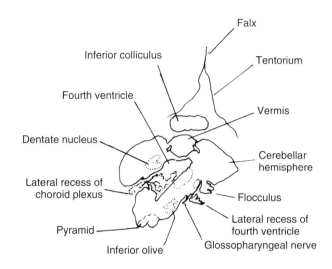

Falx

Inferior colliculus

Tentorium

Fourth ventricle

Vermis

Dentate nucleus

Cerebellar hemisphere

Lateral recess of choroid plexus

Flocculus

Pyramid

Lateral recess of fourth ventricle

Inferior olive

Glossopharyngeal nerve

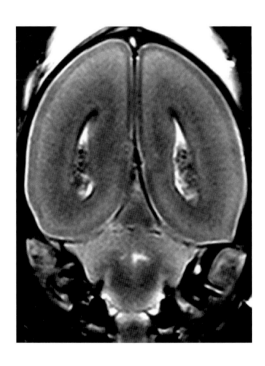

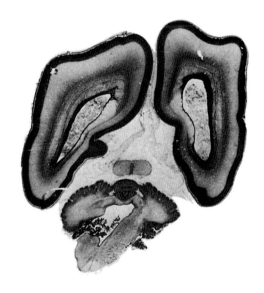

22–23 WEEKS GESTATIONAL AGE, CORONAL SECTION

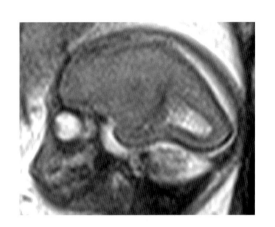

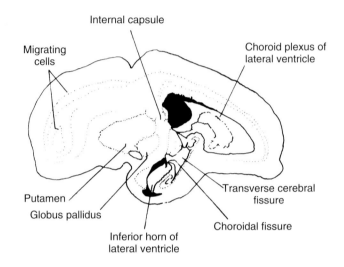

Internal capsule

Migrating cells

Choroid plexus of lateral ventricle

Putamen

Globus pallidus

Transverse cerebral fissure

Inferior horn of lateral ventricle

Choroidal fissure

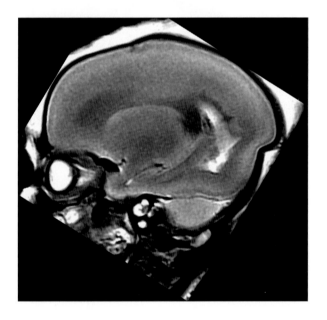

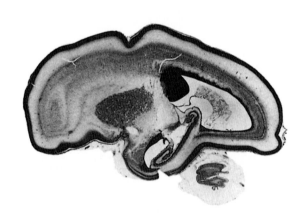

22–23 WEEKS GESTATIONAL AGE, SAGITTAL SECTION

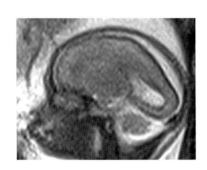

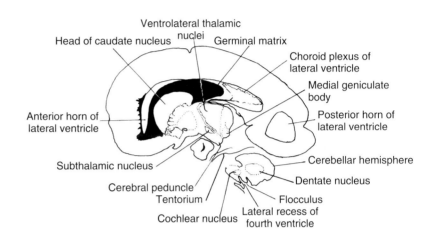

Ventrolateral thalamic
nuclei
Head of caudate nucleus   Germinal matrix

Choroid plexus of
lateral ventricle

Medial geniculate
body

Anterior horn of
lateral ventricle

Posterior horn of
lateral ventricle

Subthalamic nucleus

Cerebellar hemisphere

Dentate nucleus

Cerebral peduncle
Tentorium

Flocculus

Cochlear nucleus

Lateral recess of
fourth ventricle

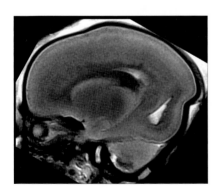

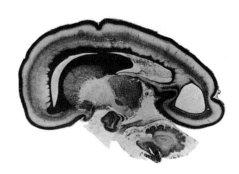

22–23 WEEKS GESTATIONAL AGE, SAGITTAL SECTION

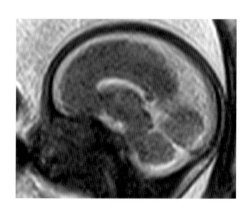

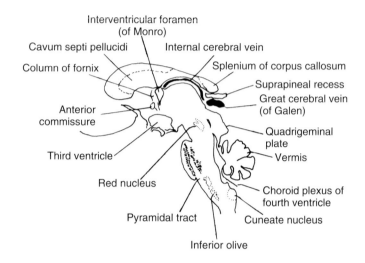

Interventricular foramen
(of Monro)

Cavum septi pellucidi

Column of fornix

Anterior
commissure

Third ventricle

Red nucleus

Pyramidal tract

Inferior olive

Internal cerebral vein

Splenium of corpus callosum

Suprapineal recess

Great cerebral vein
(of Galen)

Quadrigeminal
plate

Vermis

Choroid plexus of
fourth ventricle

Cuneate nucleus

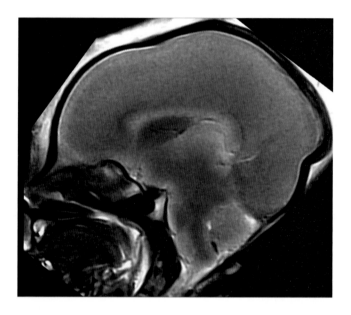

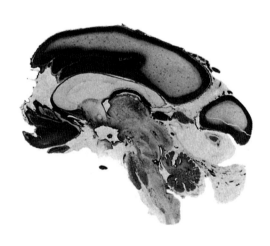

22–23 WEEKS GESTATIONAL AGE, SAGITTAL SECTION

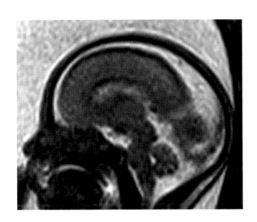

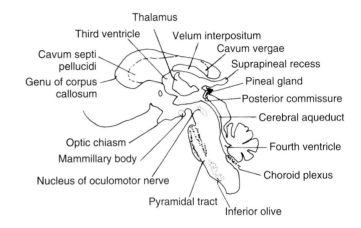

Thalamus

Third ventricle — Velum interpositum

Cavum septi pellucidi — Cavum vergae

Genu of corpus callosum — Suprapineal recess

— Pineal gland

— Posterior commissure

— Cerebral aqueduct

Optic chiasm — Fourth ventricle

Mammillary body

Nucleus of oculomotor nerve — Choroid plexus

Pyramidal tract — Inferior olive

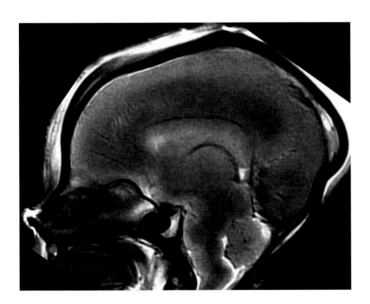

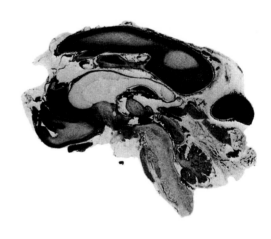

22–23 WEEKS GESTATIONAL AGE, SAGITTAL SECTION

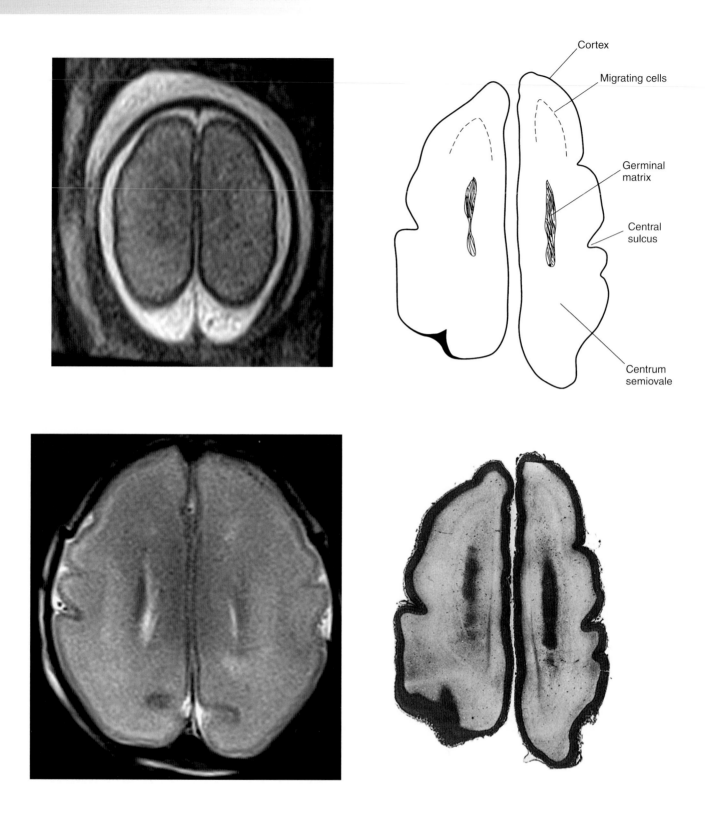

Cortex

Migrating cells

Germinal matrix

Central sulcus

Centrum semiovale

25–26 WEEKS GESTATIONAL AGE, AXIAL SECTION

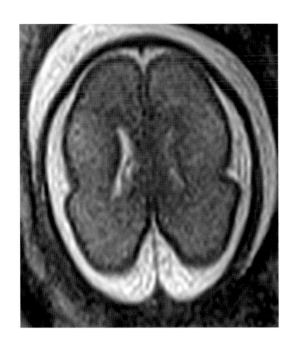

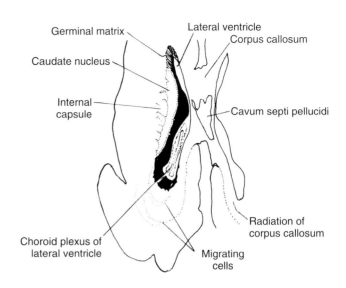

Germinal matrix

Caudate nucleus

Internal capsule

Choroid plexus of lateral ventricle

Lateral ventricle

Corpus callosum

Cavum septi pellucidi

Radiation of corpus callosum

Migrating cells

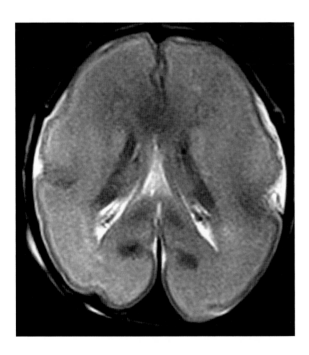

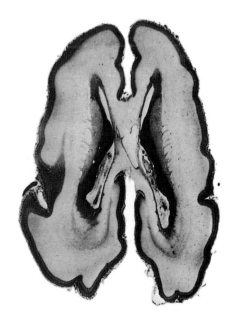

25–26 WEEKS GESTATIONAL AGE, AXIAL SECTION

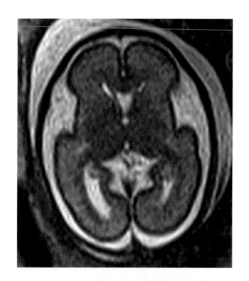

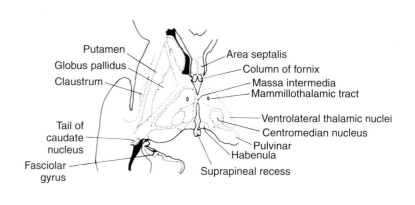

Putamen

Globus pallidus

Claustrum

Tail of
caudate
nucleus

Fasciolar
gyrus

Area septalis

Column of fornix

Massa intermedia

Mammillothalamic tract

Ventrolateral thalamic nuclei

Centromedian nucleus

Pulvinar

Habenula

Suprapineal recess

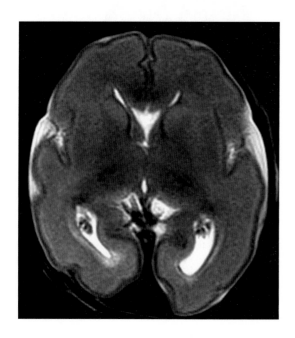

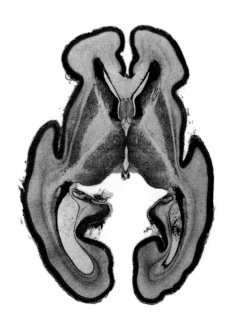

25–26 WEEKS GESTATIONAL AGE, AXIAL SECTION

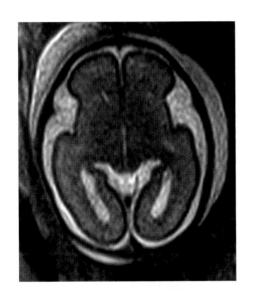

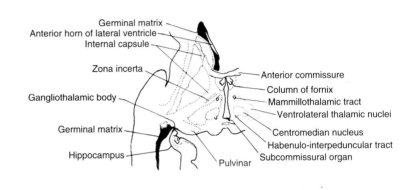

Germinal matrix
Anterior horn of lateral ventricle
Internal capsule

Zona incerta

Gangliothalamic body

Germinal matrix

Hippocampus

Pulvinar

Anterior commissure
Column of fornix
Mammillothalamic tract
Ventrolateral thalamic nuclei
Centromedian nucleus
Habenulo-interpeduncular tract
Subcommissural organ

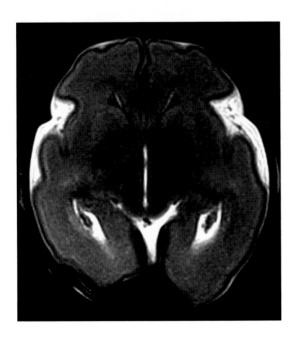

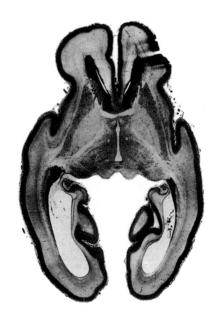

25–26 WEEKS GESTATIONAL AGE, AXIAL SECTION

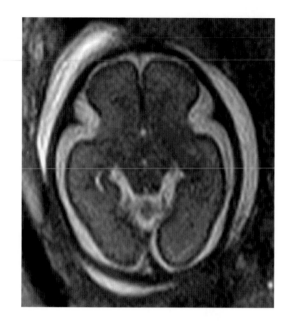

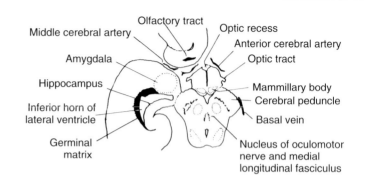

Middle cerebral artery

Amygdala

Hippocampus

Inferior horn of
lateral ventricle

Germinal
matrix

Olfactory tract

Optic recess

Anterior cerebral artery

Optic tract

Mammillary body

Cerebral peduncle

Basal vein

Nucleus of oculomotor
nerve and medial
longitudinal fasciculus

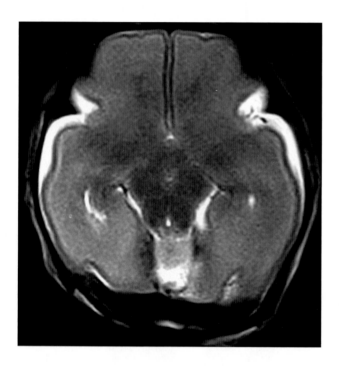

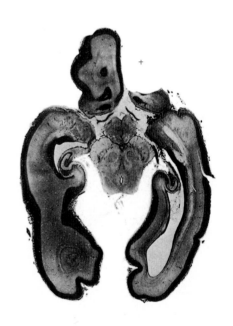

25–26 WEEKS GESTATIONAL AGE, AXIAL SECTION

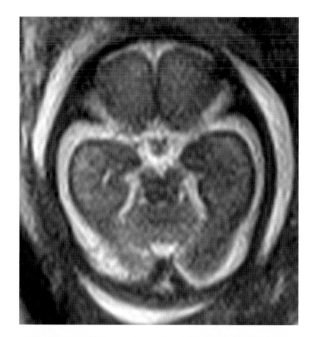

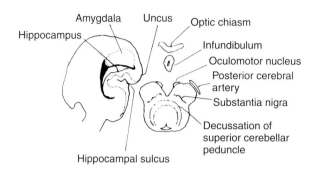

Amygdala   Uncus   Optic chiasm

Hippocampus

Infundibulum

Oculomotor nucleus

Posterior cerebral artery

Substantia nigra

Decussation of superior cerebellar peduncle

Hippocampal sulcus

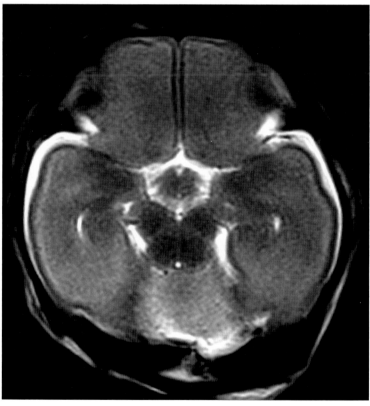

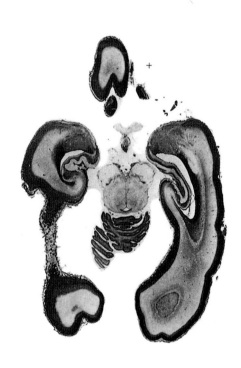

25–26 WEEKS GESTATIONAL AGE, AXIAL SECTION

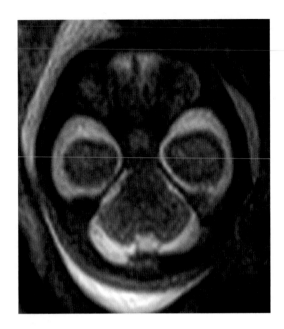

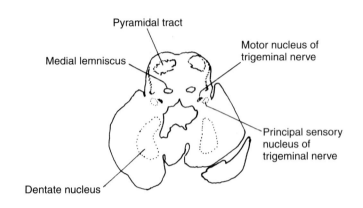

Pyramidal tract

Medial lemniscus

Motor nucleus of
trigeminal nerve

Principal sensory
nucleus of
trigeminal nerve

Dentate nucleus

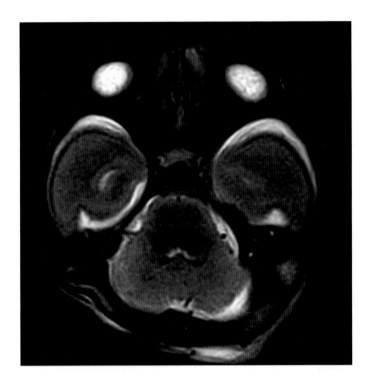

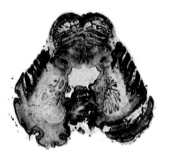

25–26 WEEKS GESTATIONAL AGE, AXIAL SECTION

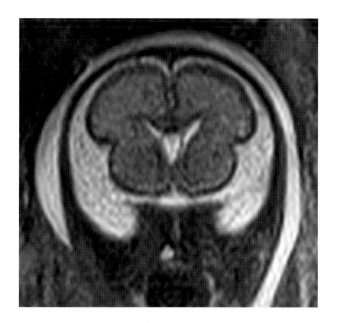

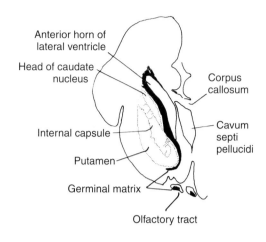

Anterior horn of
lateral ventricle

Head of caudate
nucleus

Corpus
callosum

Internal capsule

Cavum
septi
pellucidi

Putamen

Germinal matrix

Olfactory tract

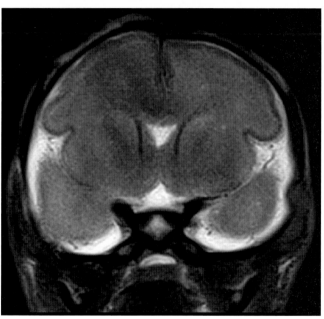

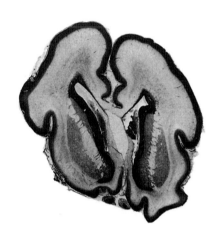

25–26 WEEKS GESTATIONAL AGE, CORONAL SECTION

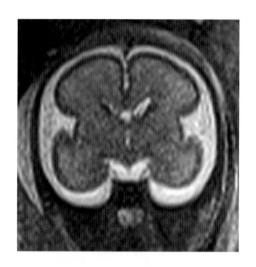

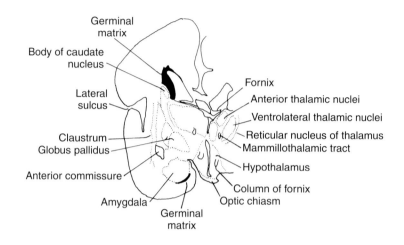

Germinal matrix

Body of caudate nucleus

Lateral sulcus

Claustrum

Globus pallidus

Anterior commissure

Amygdala

Germinal matrix

Fornix

Anterior thalamic nuclei

Ventrolateral thalamic nuclei

Reticular nucleus of thalamus

Mammillothalamic tract

Hypothalamus

Column of fornix

Optic chiasm

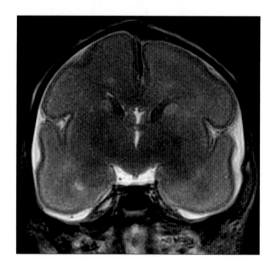

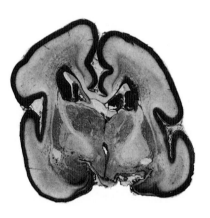

25–26 WEEKS GESTATIONAL AGE, CORONAL SECTION

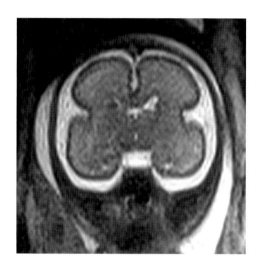

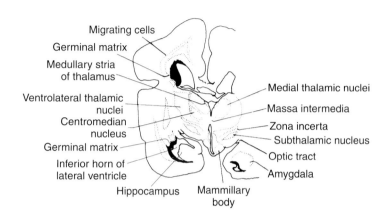

Migrating cells
Germinal matrix
Medullary stria
of thalamus
Ventrolateral thalamic
nuclei
Centromedian
nucleus
Germinal matrix
Inferior horn of
lateral ventricle
Hippocampus
Mammillary
body
Medial thalamic nuclei
Massa intermedia
Zona incerta
Subthalamic nucleus
Optic tract
Amygdala

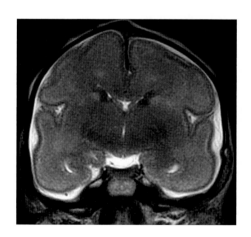

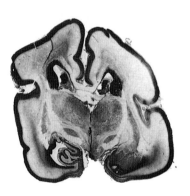

25–26 WEEKS GESTATIONAL AGE, CORONAL SECTION

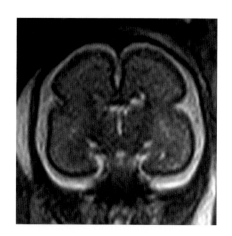

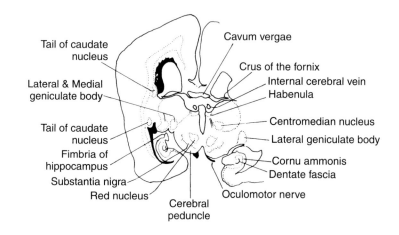

Tail of caudate nucleus

Lateral & Medial geniculate body

Tail of caudate nucleus

Fimbria of hippocampus

Substantia nigra

Red nucleus

Cerebral peduncle

Cavum vergae

Crus of the fornix

Internal cerebral vein

Habenula

Centromedian nucleus

Lateral geniculate body

Cornu ammonis

Dentate fascia

Oculomotor nerve

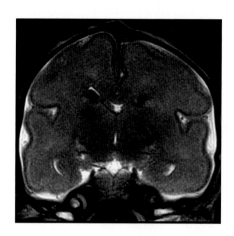

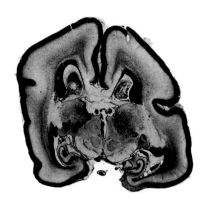

25–26 WEEKS GESTATIONAL AGE, CORONAL SECTION

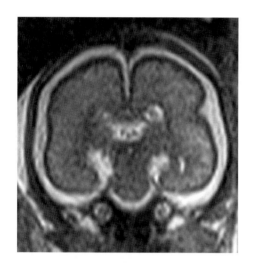

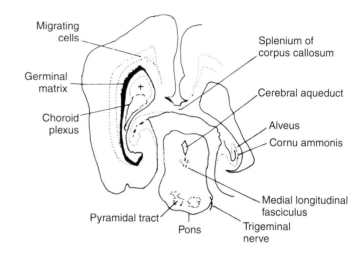

Migrating
cells

Germinal
matrix

Choroid
plexus

Pyramidal tract

Pons

Splenium of
corpus callosum

Cerebral aqueduct

Alveus

Cornu ammonis

Medial longitudinal
fasciculus

Trigeminal
nerve

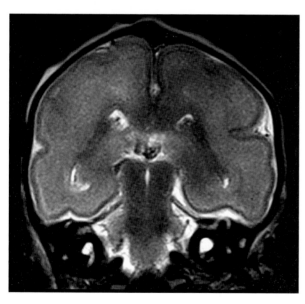

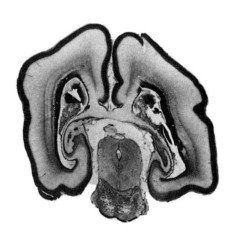

25–26 WEEKS GESTATIONAL AGE, CORONAL SECTION

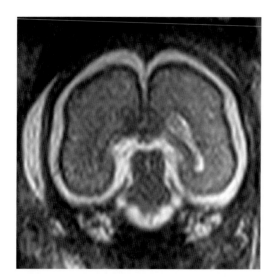

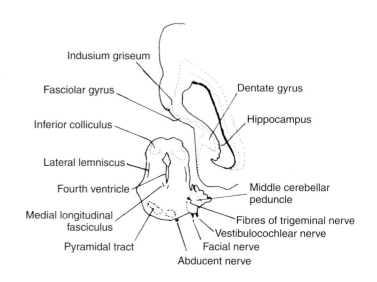

Indusium griseum

Fasciolar gyrus

Dentate gyrus

Inferior colliculus

Hippocampus

Lateral lemniscus

Fourth ventricle

Middle cerebellar peduncle

Medial longitudinal fasciculus

Fibres of trigeminal nerve

Vestibulocochlear nerve

Pyramidal tract

Facial nerve

Abducent nerve

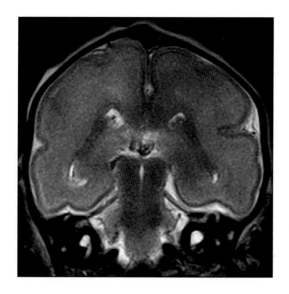

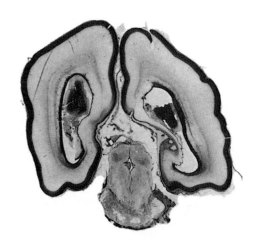

25–26 WEEKS GESTATIONAL AGE, CORONAL SECTION

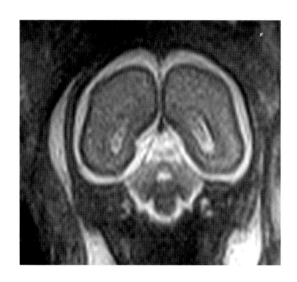

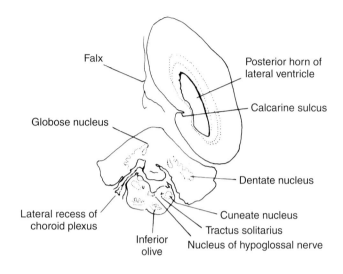

Falx

Posterior horn of
lateral ventricle

Calcarine sulcus

Globose nucleus

Dentate nucleus

Lateral recess of
choroid plexus

Cuneate nucleus

Tractus solitarius

Inferior
olive

Nucleus of hypoglossal nerve

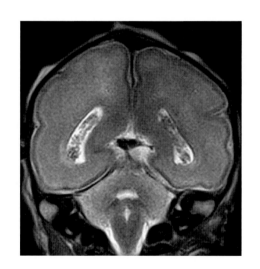

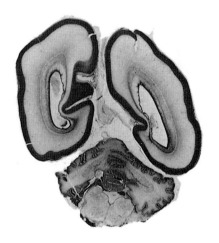

25–26 WEEKS GESTATIONAL AGE, CORONAL SECTION

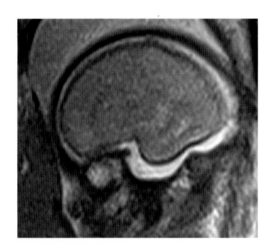

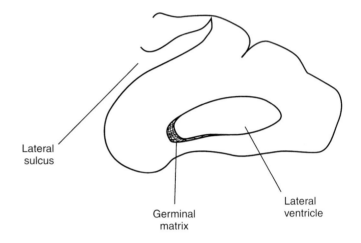

Lateral
sulcus

Germinal
matrix

Lateral
ventricle

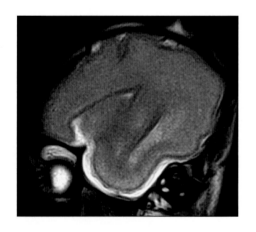

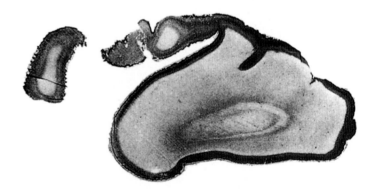

25–26 WEEKS GESTATIONAL AGE, SAGITTAL SECTION

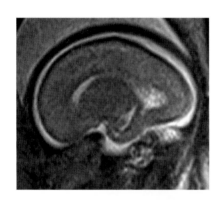

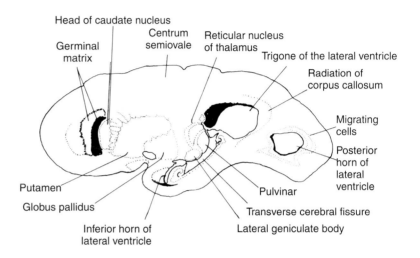

Head of caudate nucleus
Centrum semiovale
Reticular nucleus of thalamus
Trigone of the lateral ventricle
Germinal matrix
Radiation of corpus callosum
Migrating cells
Posterior horn of lateral ventricle
Putamen
Globus pallidus
Pulvinar
Transverse cerebral fissure
Lateral geniculate body
Inferior horn of lateral ventricle

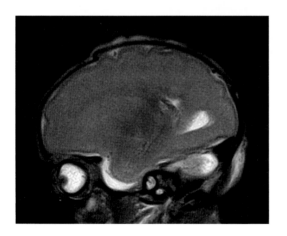

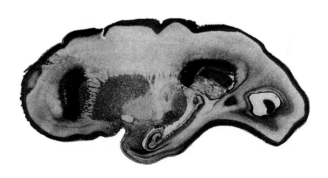

25–26 WEEKS GESTATIONAL AGE, SAGITTAL SECTION

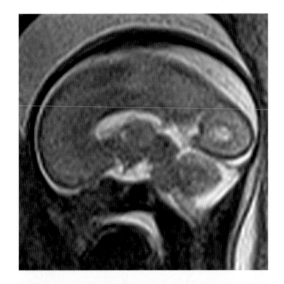

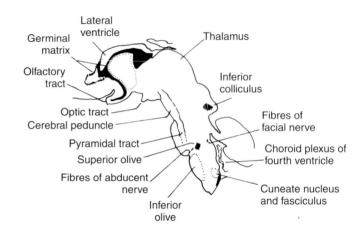

Lateral
ventricle

Germinal
matrix

Thalamus

Olfactory
tract

Inferior
colliculus

Optic tract

Cerebral peduncle

Fibres of
facial nerve

Pyramidal tract

Superior olive

Choroid plexus of
fourth ventricle

Fibres of abducent
nerve

Cuneate nucleus
and fasciculus

Inferior
olive

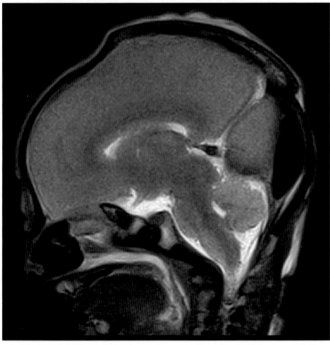

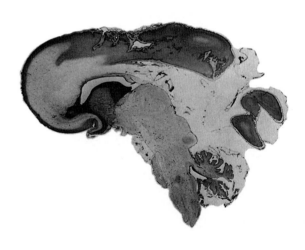

25–26 WEEKS GESTATIONAL AGE, SAGITTAL SECTION

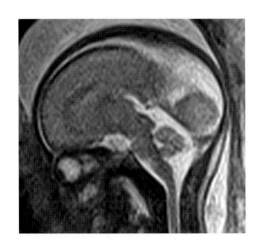

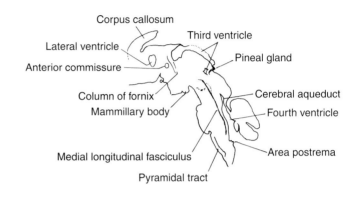

Corpus callosum

Third ventricle

Lateral ventricle

Pineal gland

Anterior commissure

Cerebral aqueduct

Column of fornix

Fourth ventricle

Mammillary body

Medial longitudinal fasciculus

Area postrema

Pyramidal tract

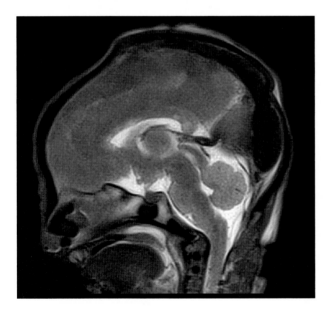

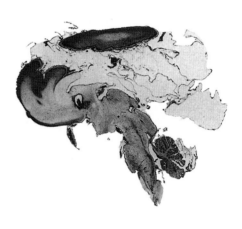

25–26 WEEKS GESTATIONAL AGE, SAGITTAL SECTION

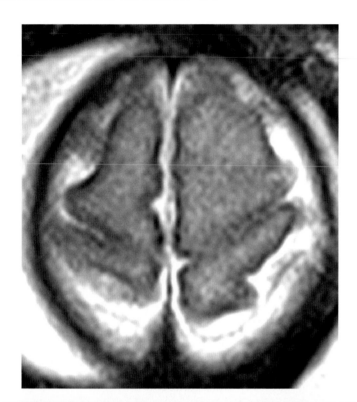

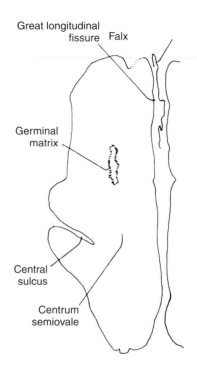

Great longitudinal fissure   Falx

Germinal matrix

Central sulcus

Centrum semiovale

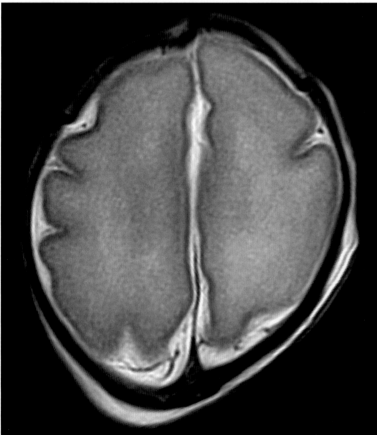

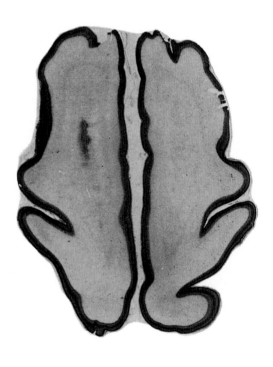

28–29 WEEKS GESTATIONAL AGE, AXIAL SECTION

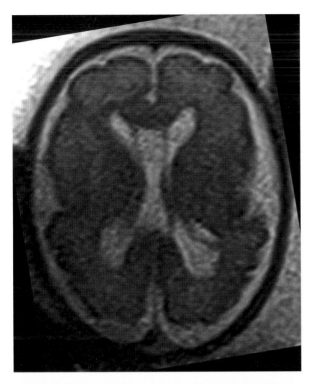

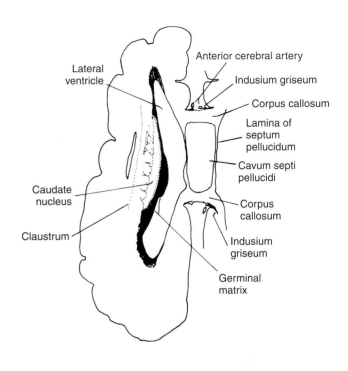

Lateral ventricle

Anterior cerebral artery

Indusium griseum

Corpus callosum

Lamina of septum pellucidum

Cavum septi pellucidi

Corpus callosum

Indusium griseum

Caudate nucleus

Claustrum

Germinal matrix

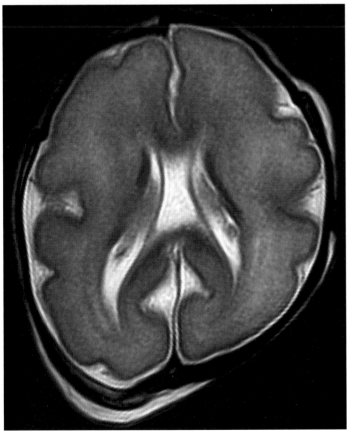

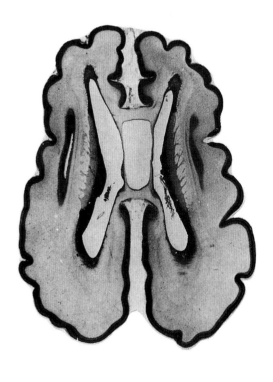

28–29 WEEKS GESTATIONAL AGE, AXIAL SECTION

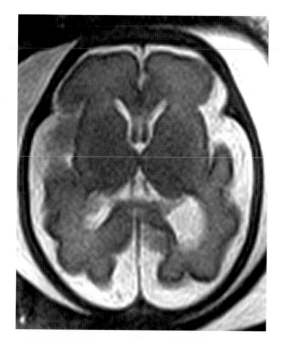

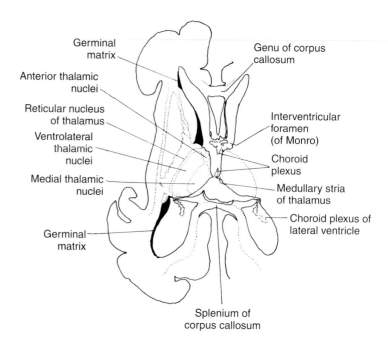

Germinal matrix

Anterior thalamic nuclei

Reticular nucleus of thalamus

Ventrolateral thalamic nuclei

Medial thalamic nuclei

Germinal matrix

Genu of corpus callosum

Interventricular foramen (of Monro)

Choroid plexus

Medullary stria of thalamus

Choroid plexus of lateral ventricle

Splenium of corpus callosum

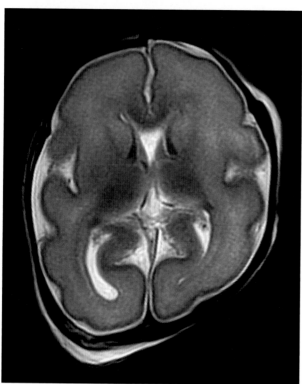

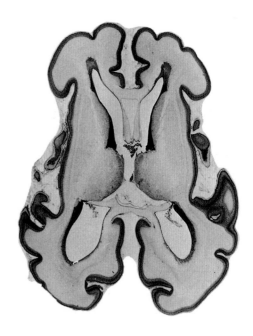

28–29 WEEKS GESTATIONAL AGE, AXIAL SECTION

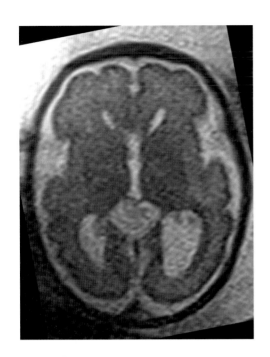

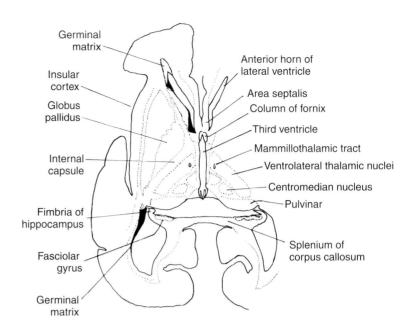

Germinal
matrix

Insular
cortex

Globus
pallidus

Internal
capsule

Fimbria of
hippocampus

Fasciolar
gyrus

Germinal
matrix

Anterior horn of
lateral ventricle

Area septalis

Column of fornix

Third ventricle

Mammillothalamic tract

Ventrolateral thalamic nuclei

Centromedian nucleus

Pulvinar

Splenium of
corpus callosum

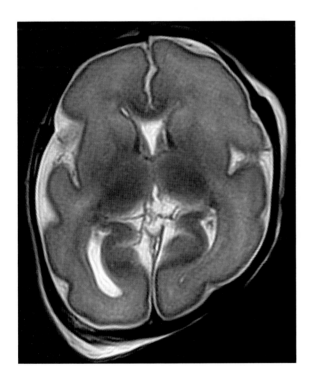

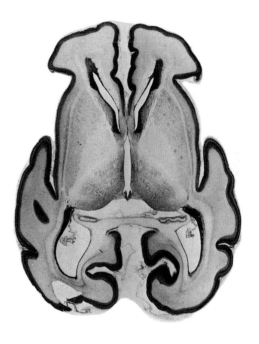

28–29 WEEKS GESTATIONAL AGE, AXIAL SECTION

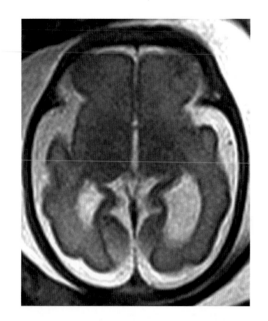

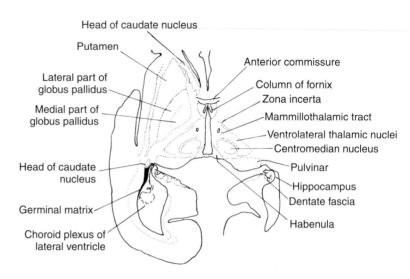

Head of caudate nucleus

Putamen

Lateral part of
globus pallidus

Medial part of
globus pallidus

Anterior commissure

Column of fornix

Zona incerta

Mammillothalamic tract

Ventrolateral thalamic nuclei

Centromedian nucleus

Pulvinar

Hippocampus

Dentate fascia

Habenula

Head of caudate
nucleus

Germinal matrix

Choroid plexus of
lateral ventricle

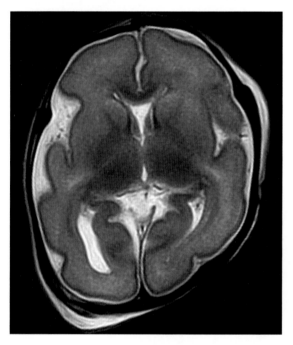

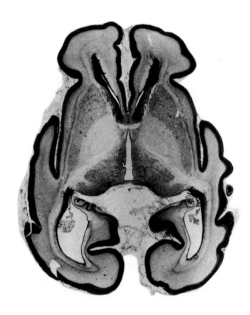

28–29 WEEKS GESTATIONAL AGE, AXIAL SECTION

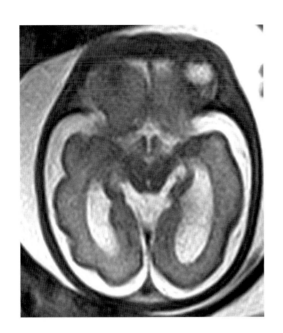

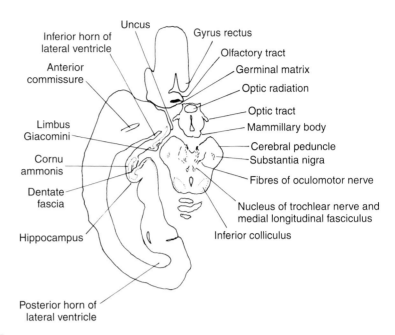

Uncus
Gyrus rectus
Inferior horn of lateral ventricle
Olfactory tract
Anterior commissure
Germinal matrix
Optic radiation
Optic tract
Limbus Giacomini
Mammillary body
Cornu ammonis
Cerebral peduncle
Substantia nigra
Dentate fascia
Fibres of oculomotor nerve
Nucleus of trochlear nerve and medial longitudinal fasciculus
Hippocampus
Inferior colliculus

Posterior horn of lateral ventricle

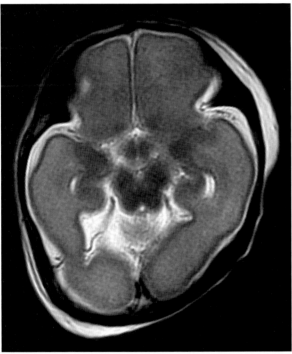

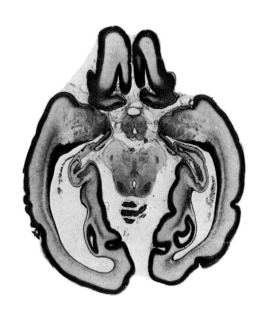

28–29 WEEKS GESTATIONAL AGE, AXIAL SECTION

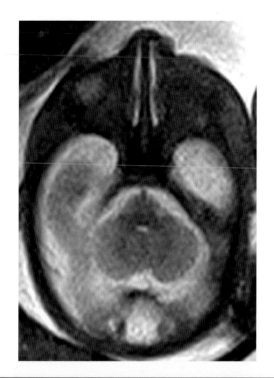

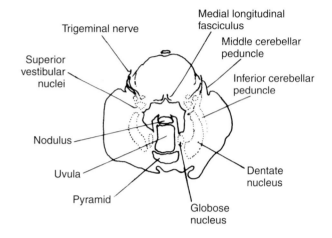

Trigeminal nerve

Medial longitudinal fasciculus

Middle cerebellar peduncle

Superior vestibular nuclei

Inferior cerebellar peduncle

Nodulus

Uvula

Dentate nucleus

Pyramid

Globose nucleus

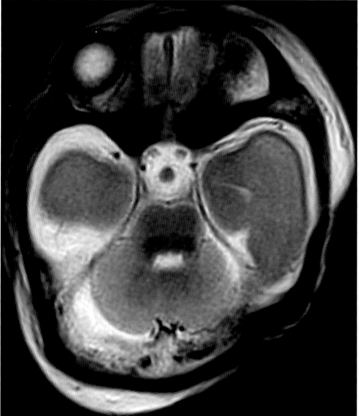

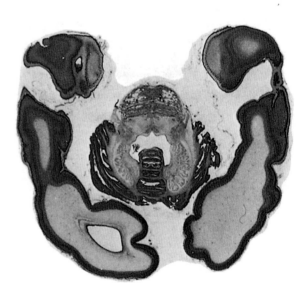

28–29 WEEKS GESTATIONAL AGE, AXIAL SECTION

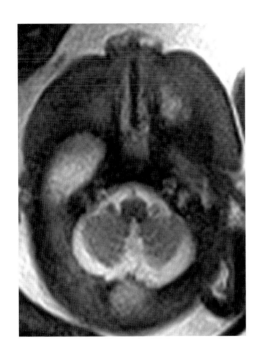

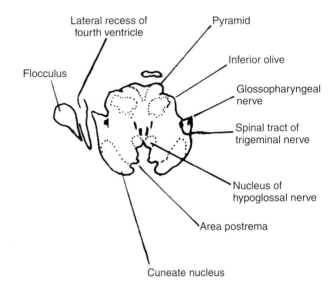

Lateral recess of
fourth ventricle

Pyramid

Flocculus

Inferior olive

Glossopharyngeal
nerve

Spinal tract of
trigeminal nerve

Nucleus of
hypoglossal nerve

Area postrema

Cuneate nucleus

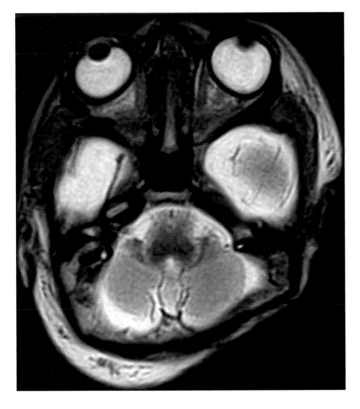

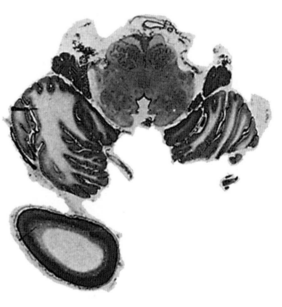

28–29 WEEKS GESTATIONAL AGE, AXIAL SECTION

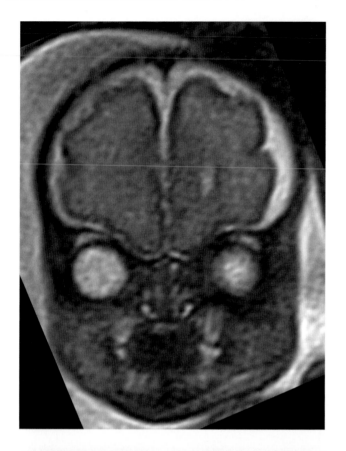

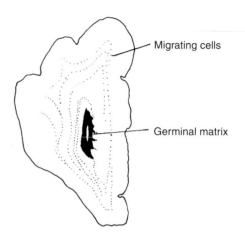

Migrating cells

Germinal matrix

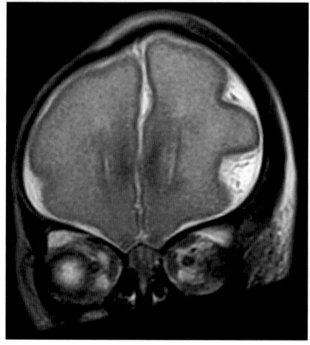

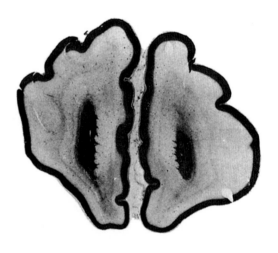

28–29 WEEKS GESTATIONAL AGE, CORONAL SECTION

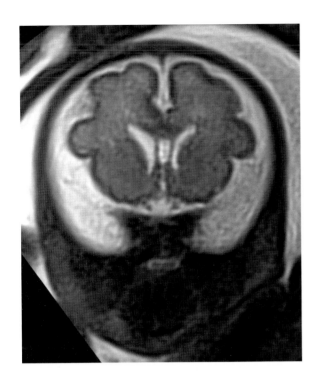

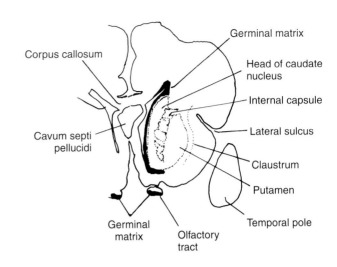

Corpus callosum

Germinal matrix

Head of caudate nucleus

Internal capsule

Lateral sulcus

Claustrum

Putamen

Temporal pole

Cavum septi pellucidi

Germinal matrix

Olfactory tract

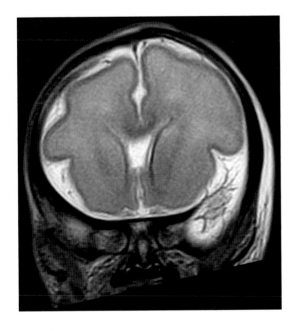

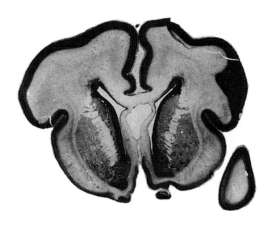

28–29 WEEKS GESTATIONAL AGE, CORONAL SECTION

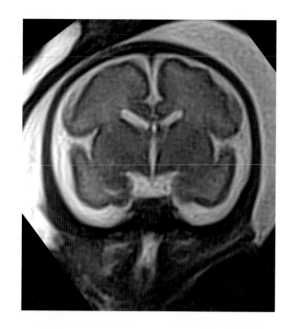

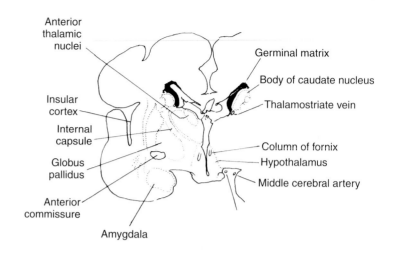

Anterior
thalamic
nuclei

Germinal matrix

Body of caudate nucleus

Insular
cortex

Thalamostriate vein

Internal
capsule

Column of fornix

Globus
pallidus

Hypothalamus

Middle cerebral artery

Anterior
commissure

Amygdala

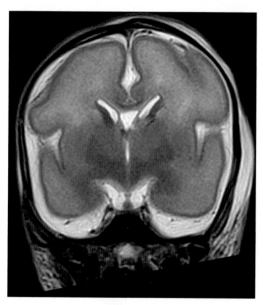

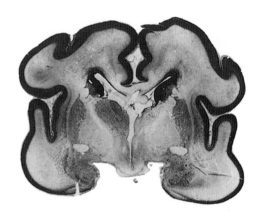

28–29 WEEKS GESTATIONAL AGE, CORONAL SECTION

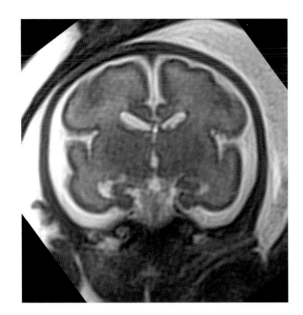

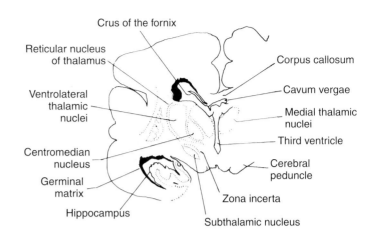

Crus of the fornix

Reticular nucleus of thalamus

Corpus callosum

Cavum vergae

Ventrolateral thalamic nuclei

Medial thalamic nuclei

Centromedian nucleus

Third ventricle

Germinal matrix

Cerebral peduncle

Hippocampus

Zona incerta

Subthalamic nucleus

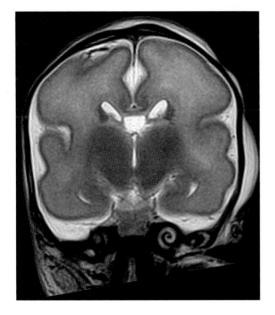

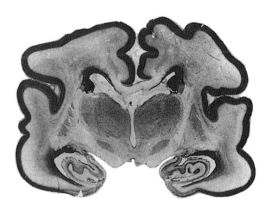

28–29 WEEKS GESTATIONAL AGE, CORONAL SECTION

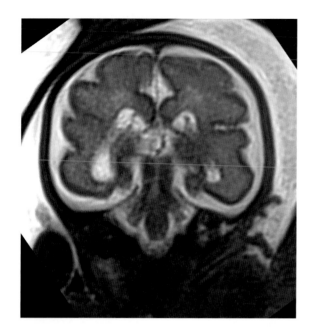

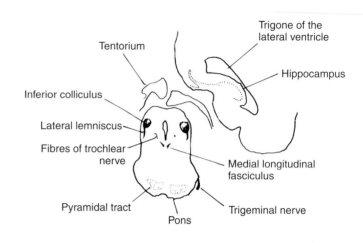

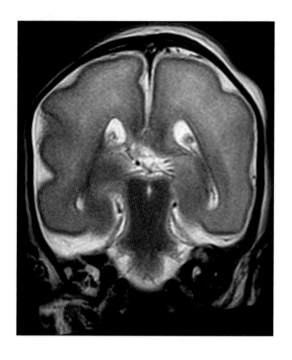

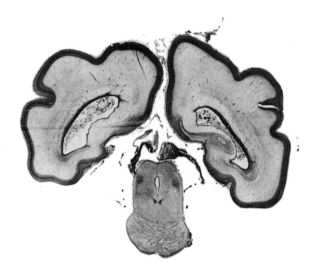

28–29 WEEKS GESTATIONAL AGE, CORONAL SECTION

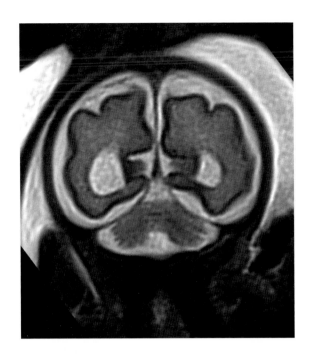

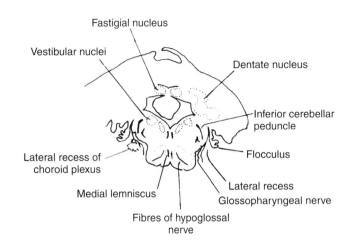

Fastigial nucleus

Vestibular nuclei

Dentate nucleus

Inferior cerebellar peduncle

Lateral recess of choroid plexus

Flocculus

Lateral recess

Medial lemniscus

Glossopharyngeal nerve

Fibres of hypoglossal nerve

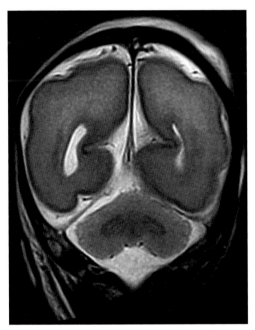

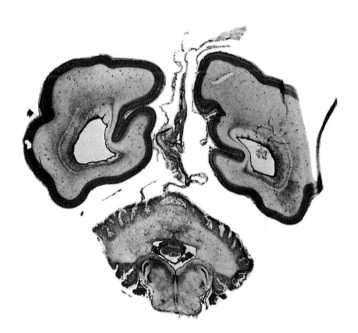

28–29 WEEKS GESTATIONAL AGE, CORONAL SECTION

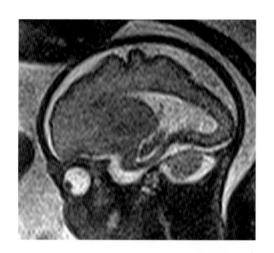

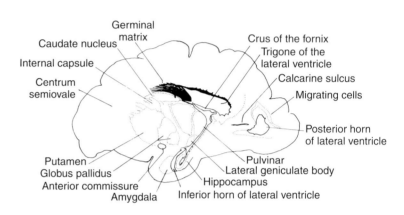

Germinal matrix

Caudate nucleus

Internal capsule

Centrum semiovale

Crus of the fornix

Trigone of the lateral ventricle

Calcarine sulcus

Migrating cells

Posterior horn of lateral ventricle

Putamen

Globus pallidus

Anterior commissure

Amygdala

Pulvinar

Lateral geniculate body

Hippocampus

Inferior horn of lateral ventricle

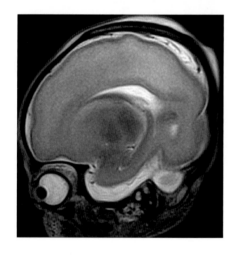

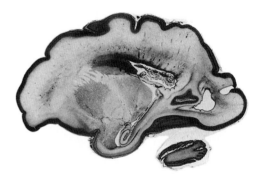

28–29 WEEKS GESTATIONAL AGE, SAGITTAL SECTION

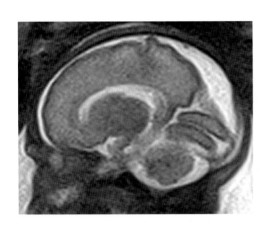

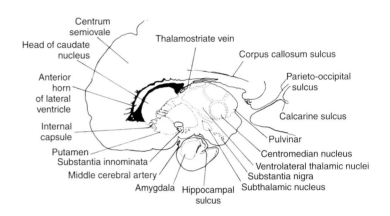

Centrum
semiovale

Head of caudate
nucleus

Thalamostriate vein

Corpus callosum sulcus

Anterior
horn
of lateral
ventricle

Parieto-occipital
sulcus

Calcarine sulcus

Internal
capsule

Pulvinar

Putamen

Centromedian nucleus

Substantia innominata

Ventrolateral thalamic nuclei

Middle cerebral artery

Substantia nigra

Amygdala Hippocampal
sulcus

Subthalamic nucleus

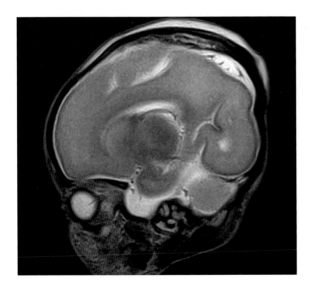

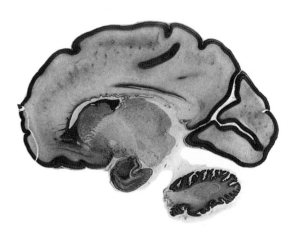

28–29 WEEKS GESTATIONAL AGE, SAGITTAL SECTION

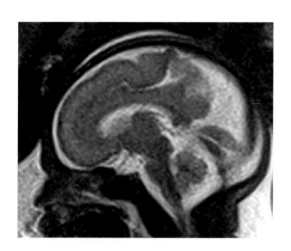

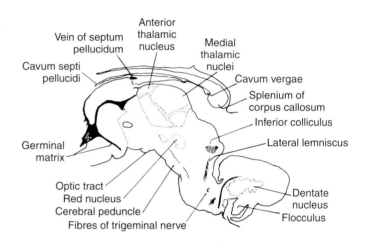

Vein of septum pellucidum

Anterior thalamic nucleus

Medial thalamic nuclei

Cavum septi pellucidi

Cavum vergae

Splenium of corpus callosum

Inferior colliculus

Germinal matrix

Lateral lemniscus

Optic tract

Red nucleus

Cerebral peduncle

Fibres of trigeminal nerve

Dentate nucleus

Flocculus

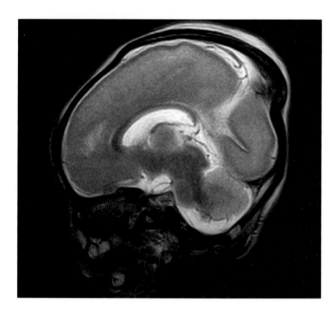

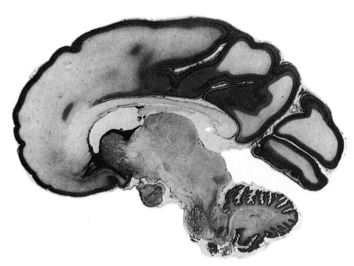

28–29 WEEKS GESTATIONAL AGE, SAGITTAL SECTION

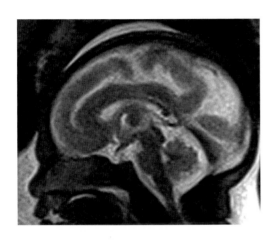

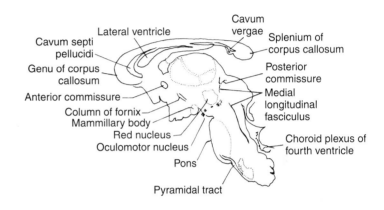

Cavum septi pellucidi
Genu of corpus callosum
Anterior commissure
Column of fornix
Mammillary body
Red nucleus
Oculomotor nucleus
Pons
Pyramidal tract
Lateral ventricle
Cavum vergae
Splenium of corpus callosum
Posterior commissure
Medial longitudinal fasciculus
Choroid plexus of fourth ventricle

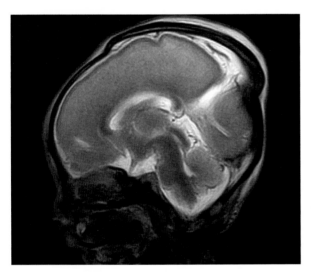

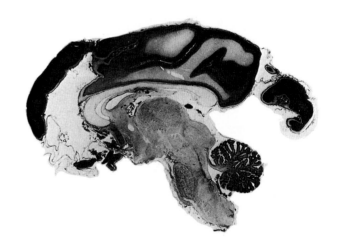

28–29 WEEKS GESTATIONAL AGE, SAGITTAL SECTION

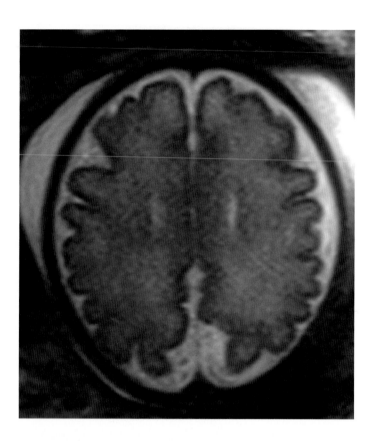

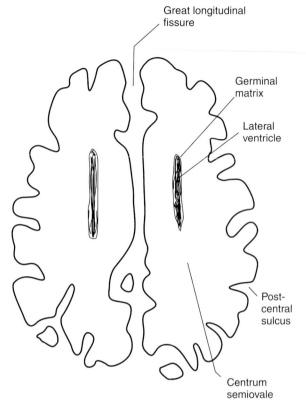

Great longitudinal fissure

Germinal matrix

Lateral ventricle

Post-central sulcus

Centrum semiovale

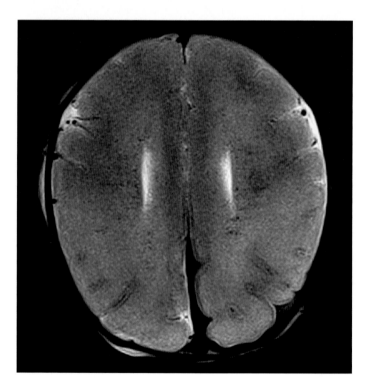

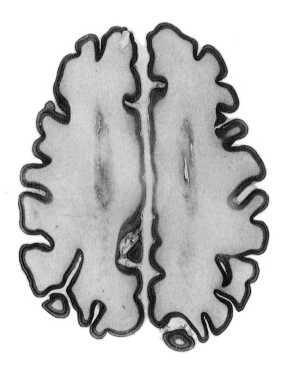

32–33 WEEKS GESTATIONAL AGE, AXIAL SECTION

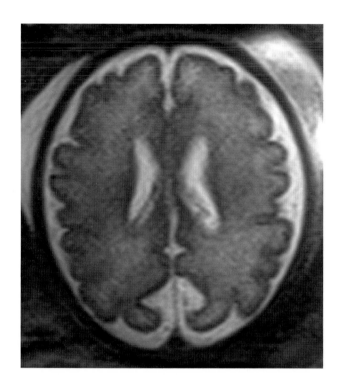

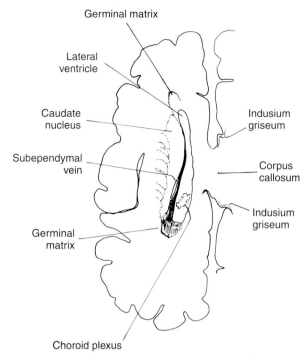

Germinal matrix

Lateral
ventricle

Caudate
nucleus

Subependymal
vein

Germinal
matrix

Indusium
griseum

Corpus
callosum

Indusium
griseum

Choroid plexus

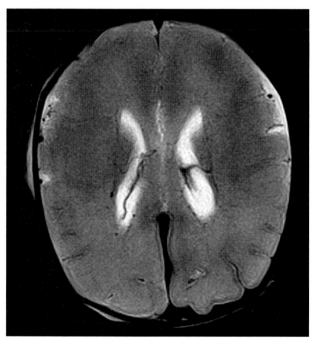

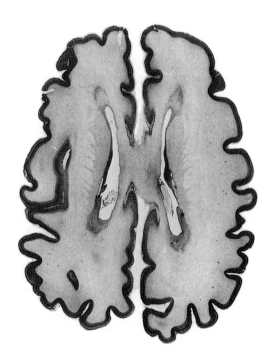

32–33 WEEKS GESTATIONAL AGE, AXIAL SECTION

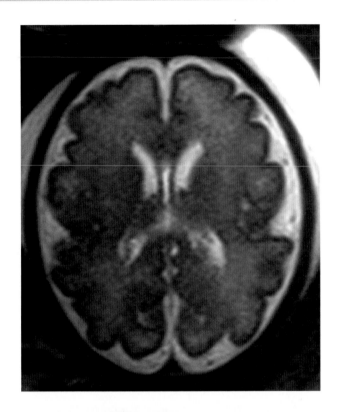

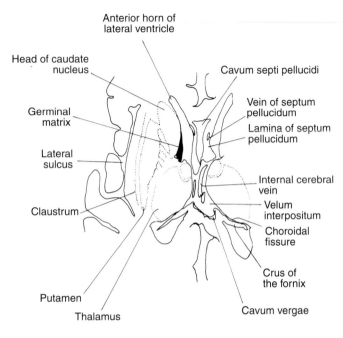

Anterior horn of
lateral ventricle

Head of caudate
nucleus

Cavum septi pellucidi

Germinal
matrix

Vein of septum
pellucidum

Lamina of septum
pellucidum

Lateral
sulcus

Internal cerebral
vein

Claustrum

Velum
interpositum

Choroidal
fissure

Putamen

Crus of
the fornix

Thalamus

Cavum vergae

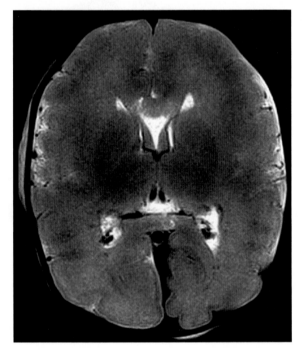

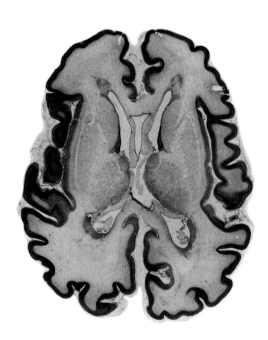

32–33 WEEKS GESTATIONAL AGE, AXIAL SECTION

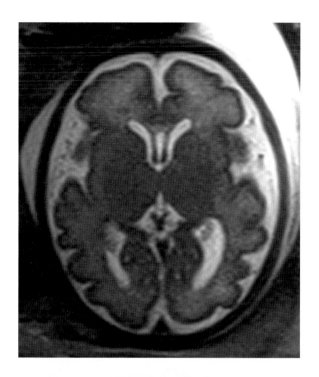

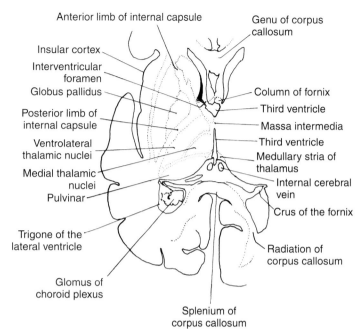

Anterior limb of internal capsule

Genu of corpus callosum

Insular cortex

Interventricular foramen

Globus pallidus

Posterior limb of internal capsule

Ventrolateral thalamic nuclei

Medial thalamic nuclei

Pulvinar

Trigone of the lateral ventricle

Glomus of choroid plexus

Column of fornix

Third ventricle

Massa intermedia

Third ventricle

Medullary stria of thalamus

Internal cerebral vein

Crus of the fornix

Radiation of corpus callosum

Splenium of corpus callosum

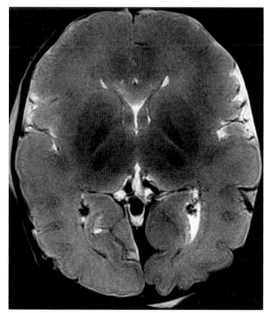

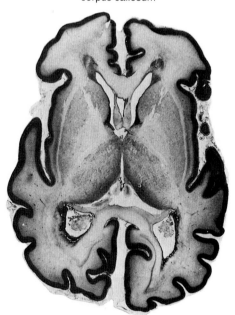

32–33 WEEKS GESTATIONAL AGE, AXIAL SECTION

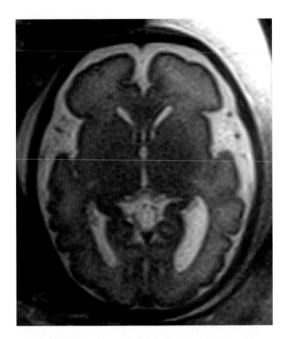

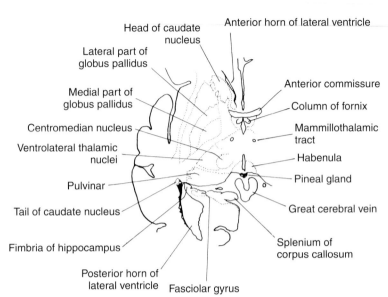

Head of caudate nucleus

Anterior horn of lateral ventricle

Lateral part of globus pallidus

Anterior commissure

Medial part of globus pallidus

Column of fornix

Centromedian nucleus

Mammillothalamic tract

Ventrolateral thalamic nuclei

Habenula

Pulvinar

Pineal gland

Tail of caudate nucleus

Great cerebral vein

Fimbria of hippocampus

Splenium of corpus callosum

Posterior horn of lateral ventricle

Fasciolar gyrus

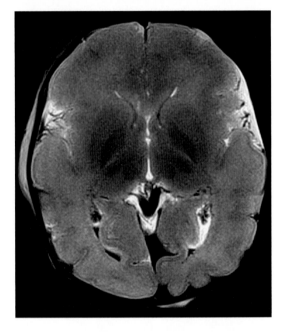

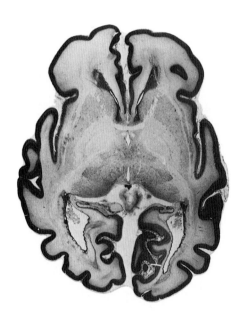

32–33 WEEKS GESTATIONAL AGE, AXIAL SECTION

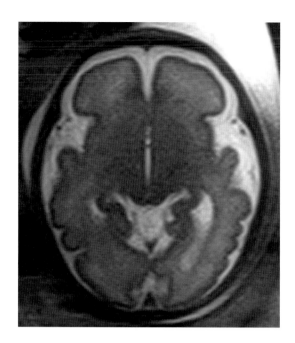

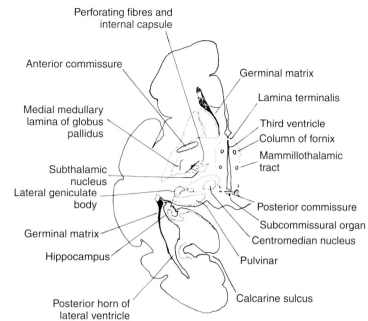

Perforating fibres and
internal capsule

Anterior commissure

Germinal matrix

Lamina terminalis

Medial medullary
lamina of globus
pallidus

Third ventricle

Column of fornix

Mammillothalamic
tract

Subthalamic
nucleus

Lateral geniculate
body

Posterior commissure

Subcommissural organ

Germinal matrix

Centromedian nucleus

Hippocampus

Pulvinar

Posterior horn of
lateral ventricle

Calcarine sulcus

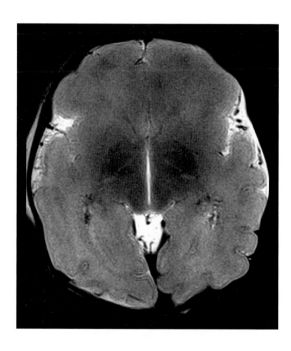

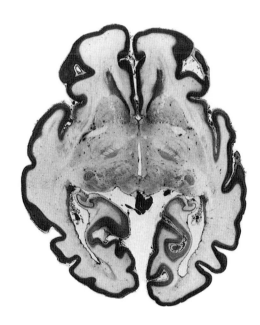

32–33 WEEKS GESTATIONAL AGE, AXIAL SECTION

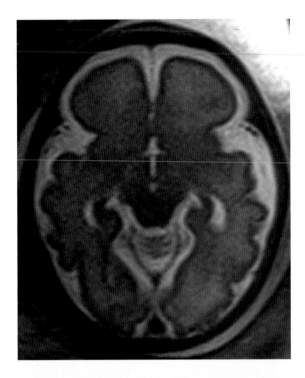

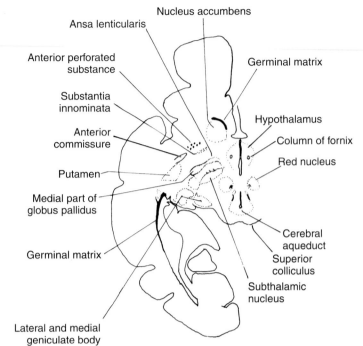

Nucleus accumbens

Ansa lenticularis

Anterior perforated substance

Germinal matrix

Substantia innominata

Hypothalamus

Anterior commissure

Column of fornix

Red nucleus

Putamen

Medial part of globus pallidus

Germinal matrix

Cerebral aqueduct

Superior colliculus

Subthalamic nucleus

Lateral and medial geniculate body

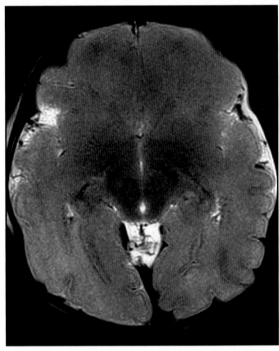

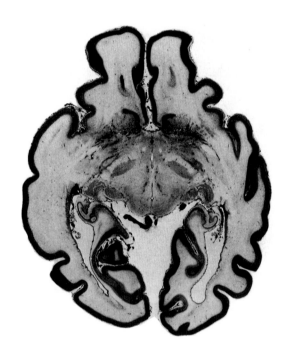

32–33 WEEKS GESTATIONAL AGE, AXIAL SECTION

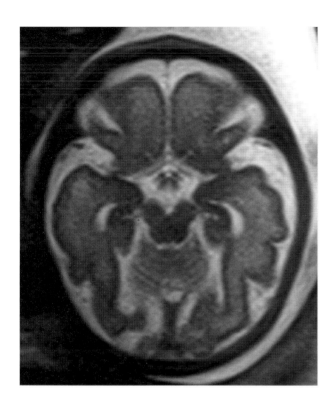

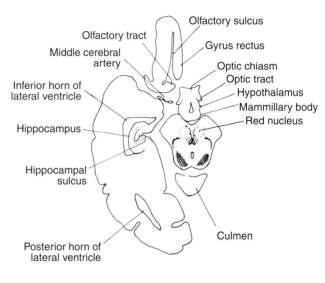

Olfactory sulcus

Olfactory tract

Middle cerebral
artery

Gyrus rectus

Optic chiasm

Optic tract

Inferior horn of
lateral ventricle

Hypothalamus

Mammillary body

Hippocampus

Red nucleus

Hippocampal
sulcus

Posterior horn of
lateral ventricle

Culmen

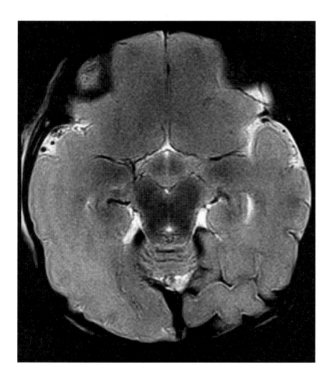

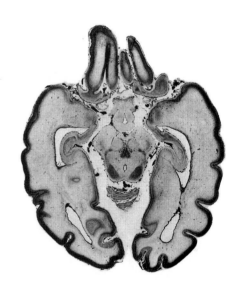

32–33 WEEKS GESTATIONAL AGE, AXIAL SECTION

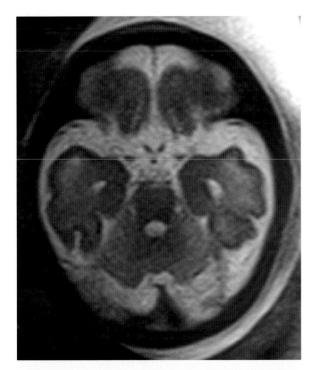

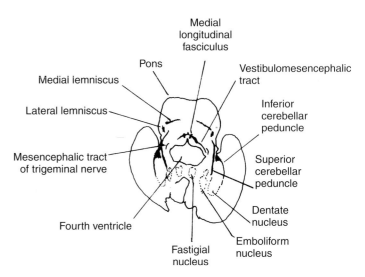

Medial
longitudinal
fasciculus

Pons

Vestibulomesencephalic
tract

Medial lemniscus

Inferior
cerebellar
peduncle

Lateral lemniscus

Mesencephalic tract
of trigeminal nerve

Superior
cerebellar
peduncle

Fourth ventricle

Dentate
nucleus

Fastigial
nucleus

Emboliform
nucleus

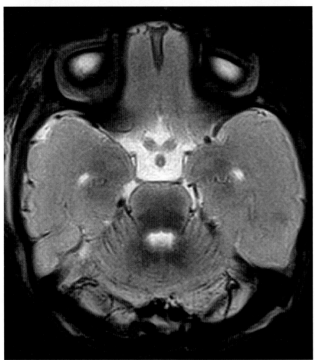

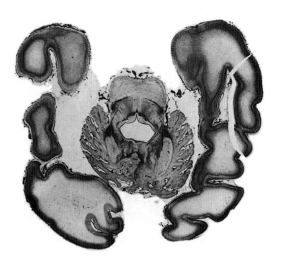

32–33 WEEKS GESTATIONAL AGE, AXIAL SECTION

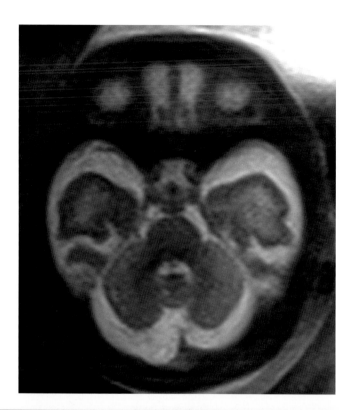

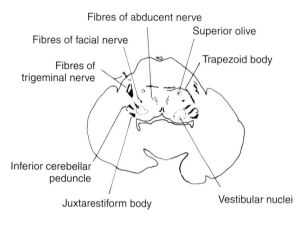

Fibres of abducent nerve

Fibres of facial nerve

Superior olive

Fibres of
trigeminal nerve

Trapezoid body

Inferior cerebellar
peduncle

Juxtarestiform body

Vestibular nuclei

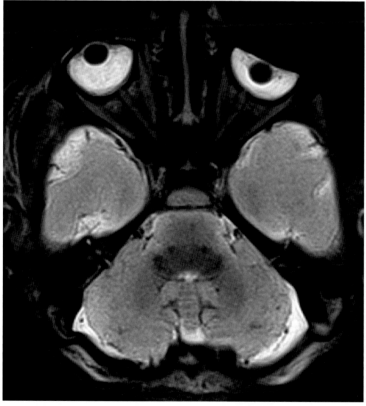

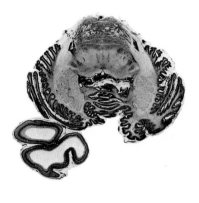

32–33 WEEKS GESTATIONAL AGE, AXIAL SECTION

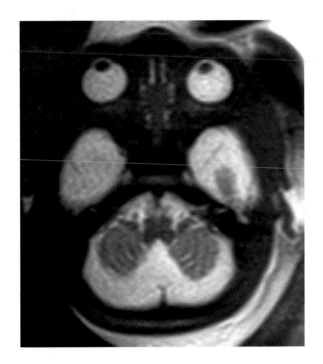

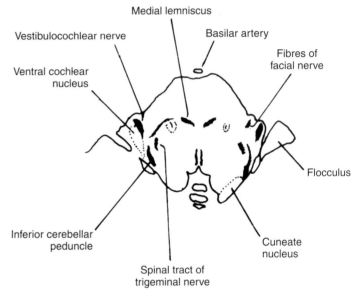

Medial lemniscus

Vestibulocochlear nerve

Basilar artery

Ventral cochlear nucleus

Fibres of facial nerve

Flocculus

Inferior cerebellar peduncle

Cuneate nucleus

Spinal tract of trigeminal nerve

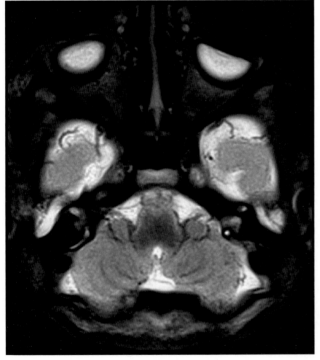

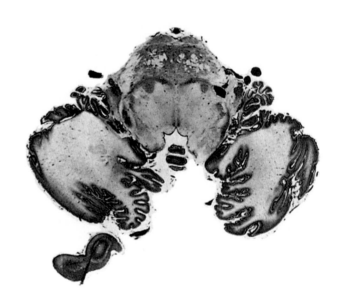

32–33 WEEKS GESTATIONAL AGE, AXIAL SECTION

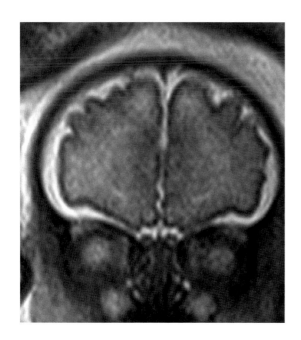

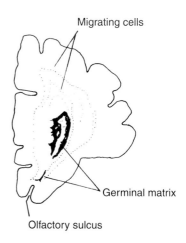

Migrating cells

Germinal matrix

Olfactory sulcus

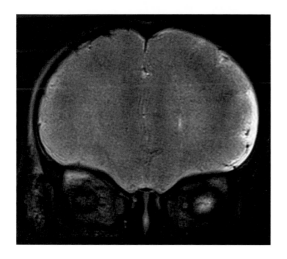

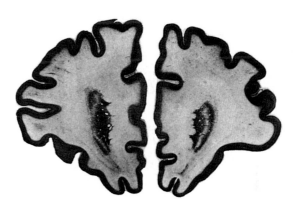

32–33 WEEKS GESTATIONAL AGE, CORONAL SECTION

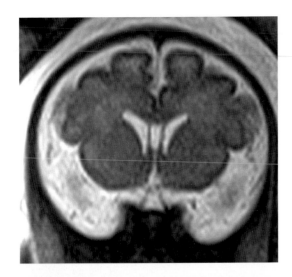

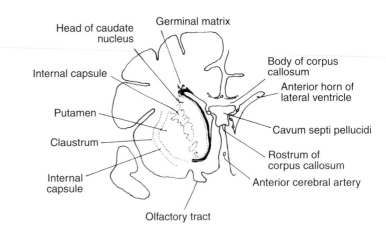

Head of caudate nucleus

Germinal matrix

Internal capsule

Body of corpus callosum

Anterior horn of lateral ventricle

Putamen

Cavum septi pellucidi

Claustrum

Rostrum of corpus callosum

Internal capsule

Anterior cerebral artery

Olfactory tract

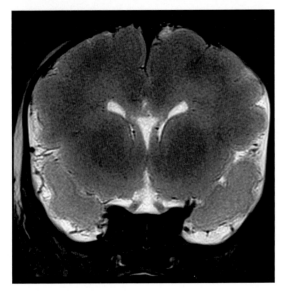

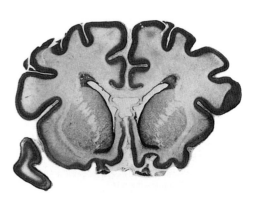

32–33 WEEKS GESTATIONAL AGE, CORONAL SECTION

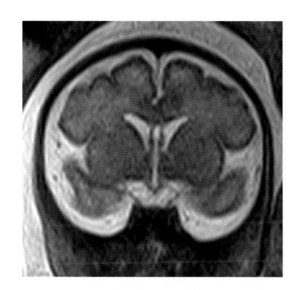

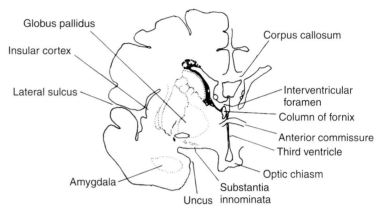

Globus pallidus

Insular cortex

Lateral sulcus

Corpus callosum

Interventricular foramen

Column of fornix

Anterior commissure

Third ventricle

Optic chiasm

Amygdala

Uncus

Substantia innominata

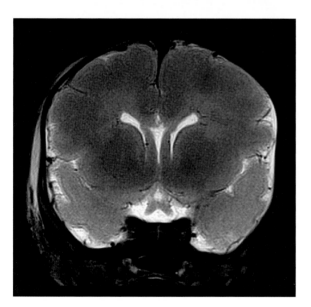

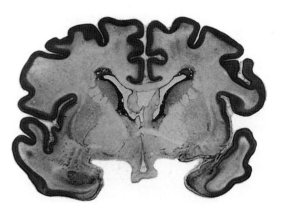

32–33 WEEKS GESTATIONAL AGE, CORONAL SECTION

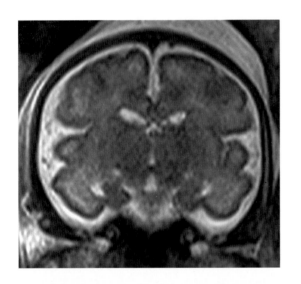

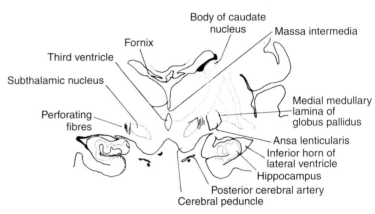

Body of caudate nucleus

Massa intermedia

Fornix

Third ventricle

Subthalamic nucleus

Medial medullary lamina of globus pallidus

Perforating fibres

Ansa lenticularis

Inferior horn of lateral ventricle

Hippocampus

Posterior cerebral artery

Cerebral peduncle

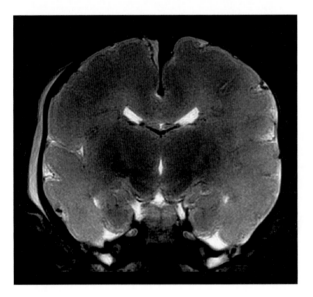

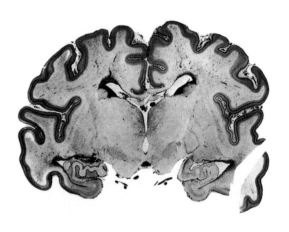

32–33 WEEKS GESTATIONAL AGE, CORONAL SECTION

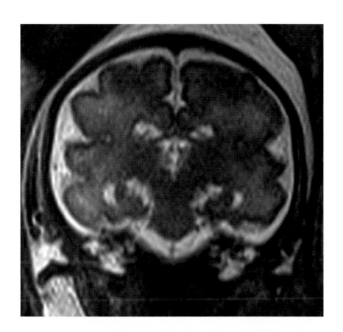

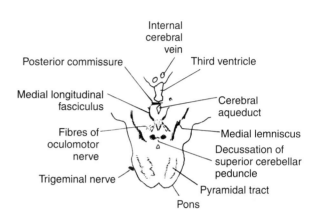

Internal cerebral vein

Third ventricle

Posterior commissure

Medial longitudinal fasciculus

Cerebral aqueduct

Fibres of oculomotor nerve

Medial lemniscus

Decussation of superior cerebellar peduncle

Trigeminal nerve

Pyramidal tract

Pons

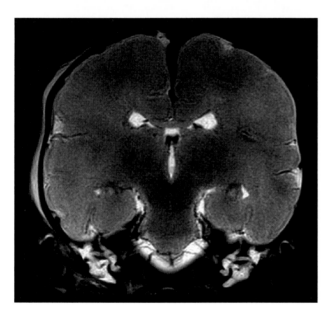

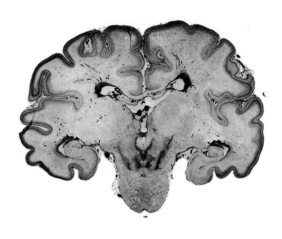

32–33 WEEKS GESTATIONAL AGE, CORONAL SECTION

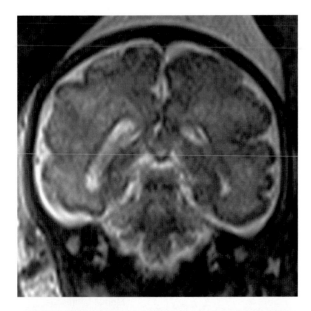

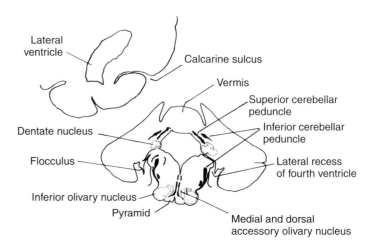

Lateral ventricle

Calcarine sulcus

Vermis

Superior cerebellar peduncle

Dentate nucleus

Inferior cerebellar peduncle

Flocculus

Lateral recess of fourth ventricle

Inferior olivary nucleus

Pyramid

Medial and dorsal accessory olivary nucleus

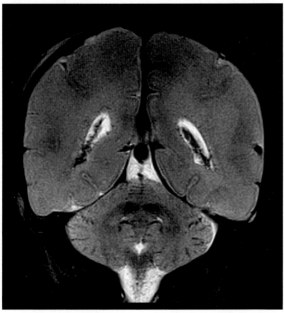

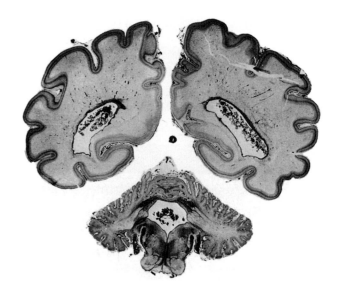

32–33 WEEKS GESTATIONAL AGE, CORONAL SECTION

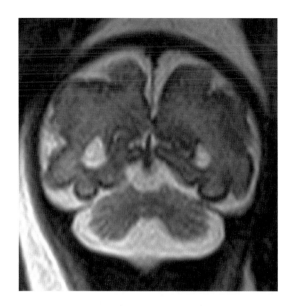

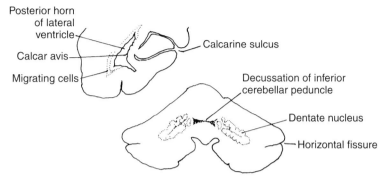

Posterior horn
of lateral
ventricle

Calcar avis

Migrating cells

Calcarine sulcus

Decussation of inferior
cerebellar peduncle

Dentate nucleus

Horizontal fissure

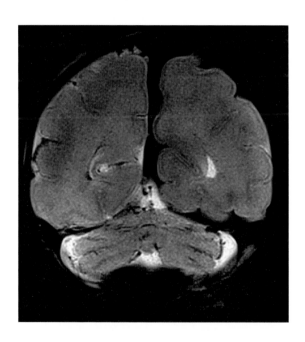

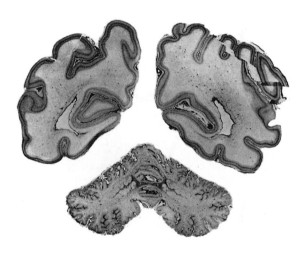

32–33 WEEKS GESTATIONAL AGE, CORONAL SECTION

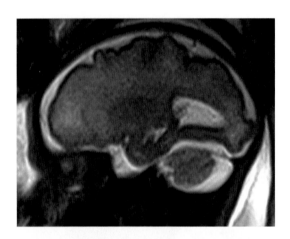

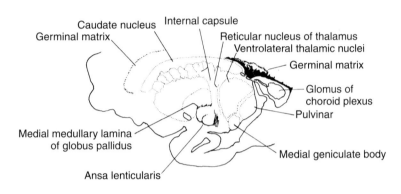

Caudate nucleus

Germinal matrix

Internal capsule

Reticular nucleus of thalamus

Ventrolateral thalamic nuclei

Germinal matrix

Glomus of choroid plexus

Pulvinar

Medial medullary lamina of globus pallidus

Ansa lenticularis

Medial geniculate body

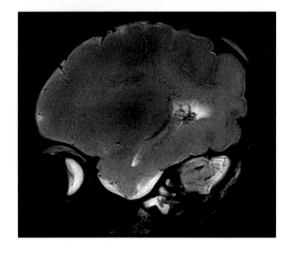

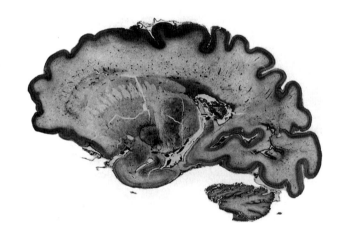

32–33 WEEKS GESTATIONAL AGE, SAGITTAL SECTION

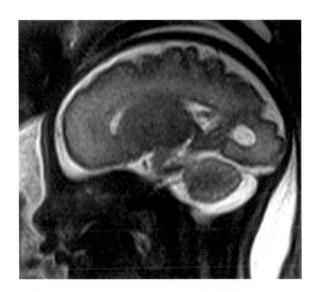

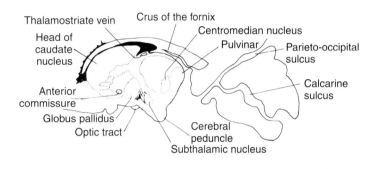

Thalamostriate vein

Head of caudate nucleus

Crus of the fornix

Centromedian nucleus

Pulvinar

Parieto-occipital sulcus

Calcarine sulcus

Anterior commissure

Globus pallidus

Optic tract

Cerebral peduncle

Subthalamic nucleus

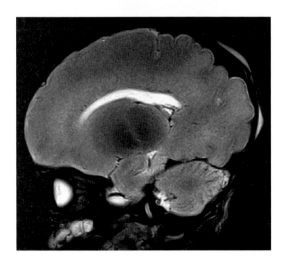

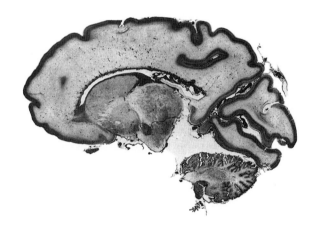

32–33 WEEKS GESTATIONAL AGE, SAGITTAL SECTION

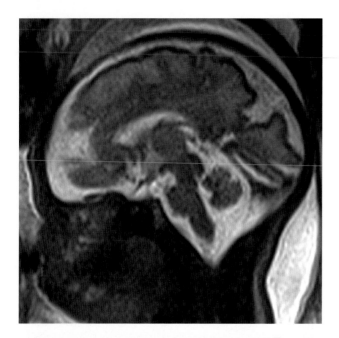

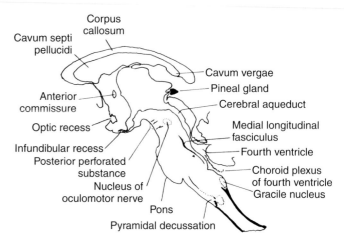

Corpus
callosum

Cavum septi
pellucidi

Cavum vergae

Anterior
commissure

Pineal gland

Cerebral aqueduct

Optic recess

Medial longitudinal
fasciculus

Infundibular recess

Fourth ventricle

Posterior perforated
substance

Choroid plexus
of fourth ventricle

Nucleus of
oculomotor nerve

Gracile nucleus

Pons

Pyramidal decussation

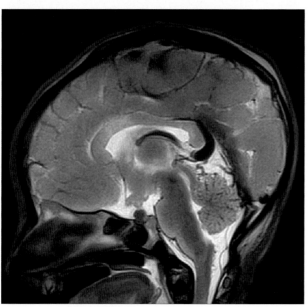

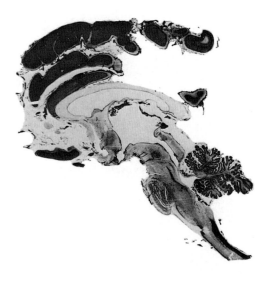

32–33 WEEKS GESTATIONAL AGE, SAGITTAL SECTION

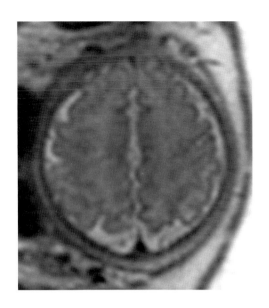

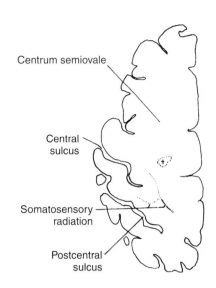

Centrum semiovale

Central
sulcus

Somatosensory
radiation

Postcentral
sulcus

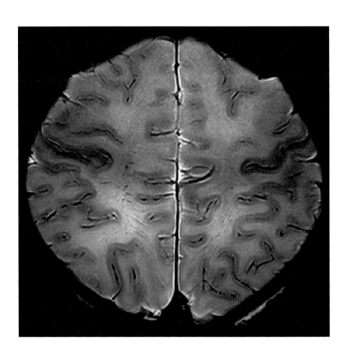

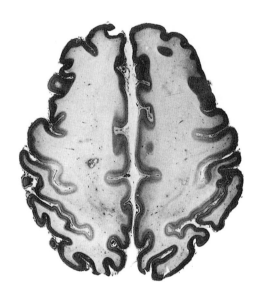

36–37 WEEKS GESTATIONAL AGE, AXIAL SECTION

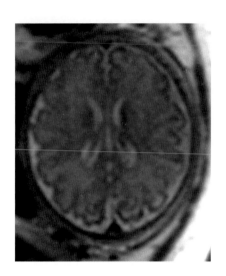

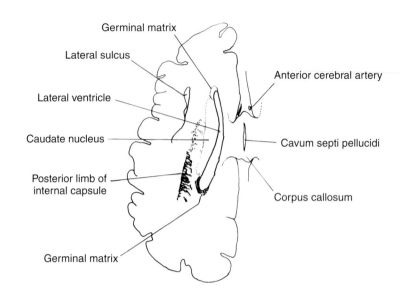

Germinal matrix

Lateral sulcus

Lateral ventricle

Caudate nucleus

Posterior limb of
internal capsule

Germinal matrix

Anterior cerebral artery

Cavum septi pellucidi

Corpus callosum

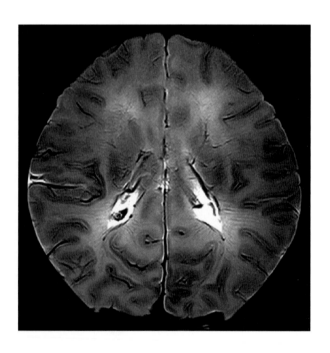

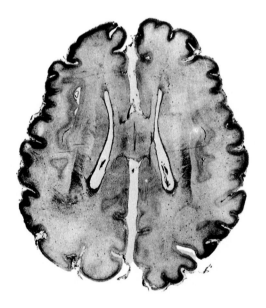

36–37 WEEKS GESTATIONAL AGE, AXIAL SECTION

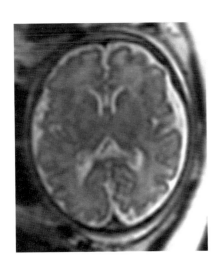

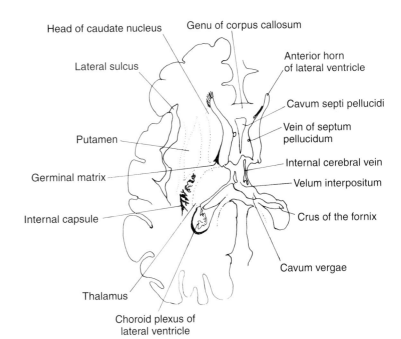

Head of caudate nucleus

Genu of corpus callosum

Lateral sulcus

Anterior horn of lateral ventricle

Cavum septi pellucidi

Putamen

Vein of septum pellucidum

Germinal matrix

Internal cerebral vein

Velum interpositum

Internal capsule

Crus of the fornix

Cavum vergae

Thalamus

Choroid plexus of lateral ventricle

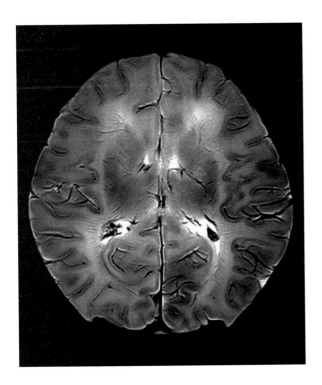

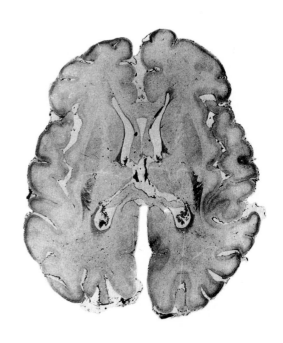

36–37 WEEKS GESTATIONAL AGE, AXIAL SECTION

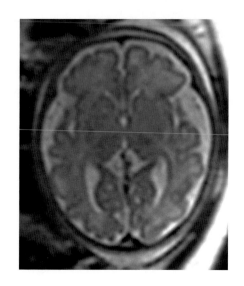

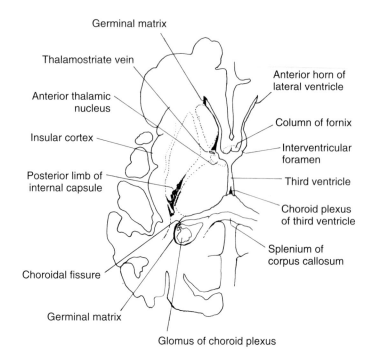

Germinal matrix

Thalamostriate vein

Anterior thalamic nucleus

Insular cortex

Posterior limb of internal capsule

Choroidal fissure

Germinal matrix

Glomus of choroid plexus

Anterior horn of lateral ventricle

Column of fornix

Interventricular foramen

Third ventricle

Choroid plexus of third ventricle

Splenium of corpus callosum

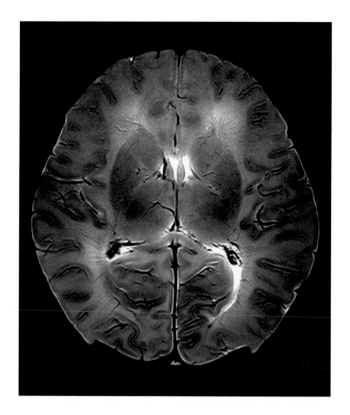

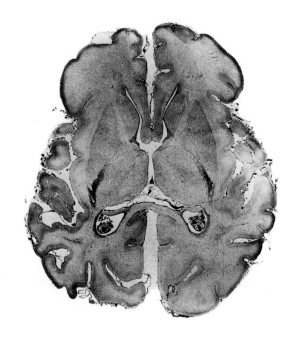

36–37 WEEKS GESTATIONAL AGE, AXIAL SECTION

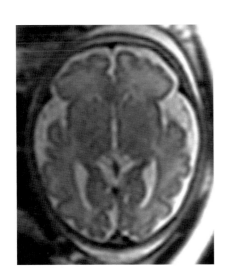

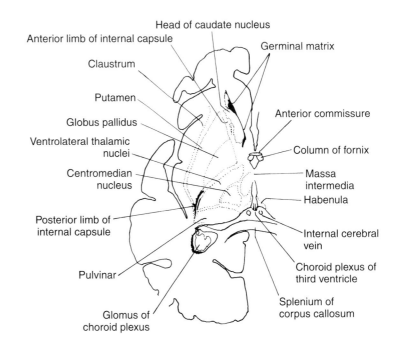

Head of caudate nucleus

Anterior limb of internal capsule

Germinal matrix

Claustrum

Putamen

Anterior commissure

Globus pallidus

Column of fornix

Ventrolateral thalamic nuclei

Massa intermedia

Centromedian nucleus

Habenula

Posterior limb of internal capsule

Internal cerebral vein

Choroid plexus of third ventricle

Pulvinar

Splenium of corpus callosum

Glomus of choroid plexus

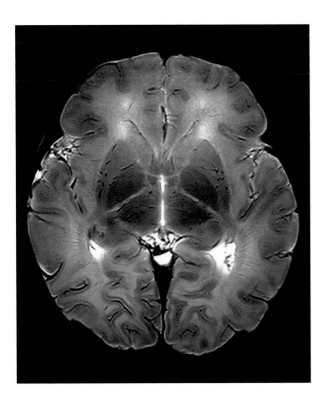

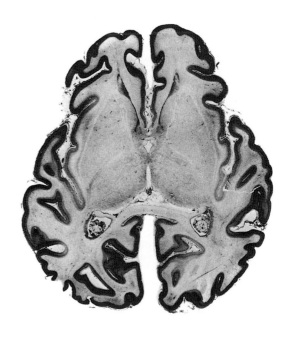

36–37 WEEKS GESTATIONAL AGE, AXIAL SECTION

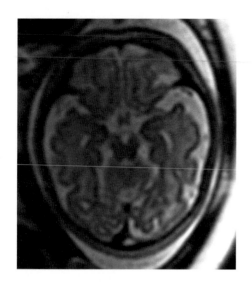

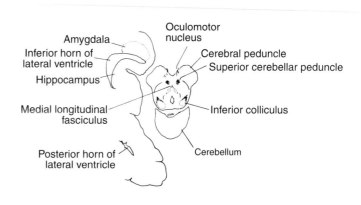

Amygdala

Inferior horn of
lateral ventricle

Hippocampus

Medial longitudinal
fasciculus

Posterior horn of
lateral ventricle

Oculomotor
nucleus

Cerebral peduncle

Superior cerebellar peduncle

Inferior colliculus

Cerebellum

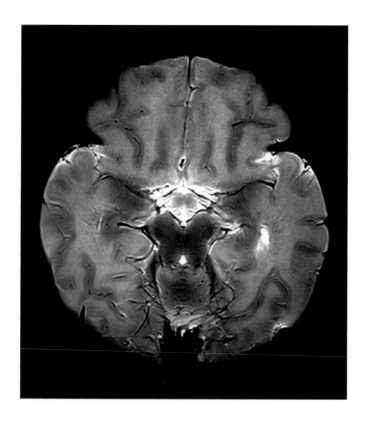

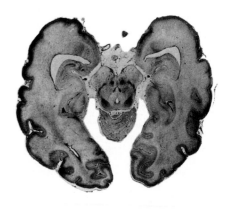

36–37 WEEKS GESTATIONAL AGE, AXIAL SECTION

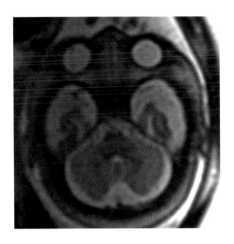

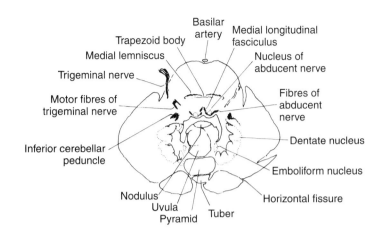

Basilar
artery
Trapezoid body
Medial longitudinal
fasciculus
Medial lemniscus
Trigeminal nerve
Nucleus of
abducent nerve
Motor fibres of
trigeminal nerve
Fibres of
abducent
nerve
Dentate nucleus
Inferior cerebellar
peduncle
Emboliform nucleus
Horizontal fissure
Nodulus
Uvula
Pyramid
Tuber

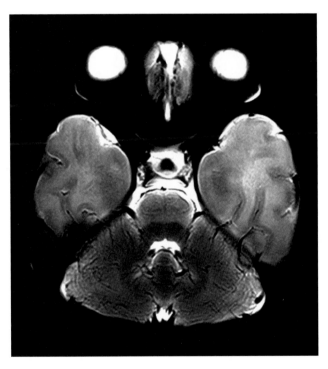

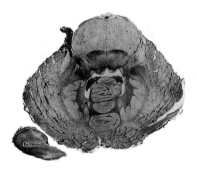

36–37 WEEKS GESTATIONAL AGE, AXIAL SECTION

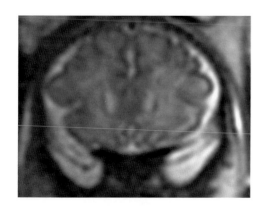

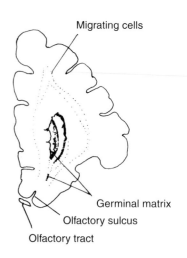

Migrating cells

Germinal matrix

Olfactory sulcus

Olfactory tract

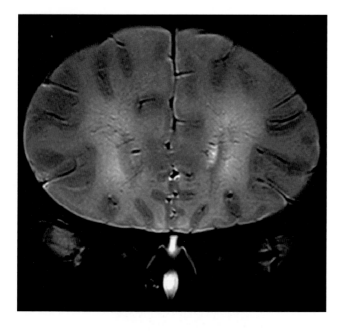

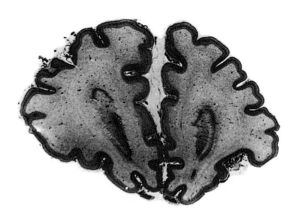

36–37 WEEKS GESTATIONAL AGE, CORONAL SECTION

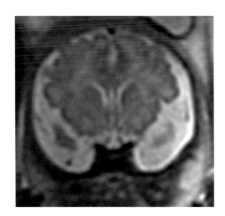

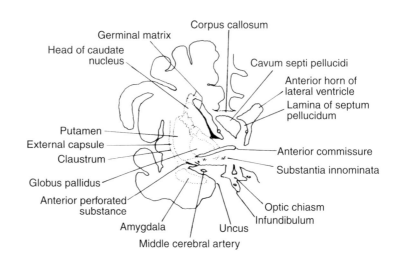

Corpus callosum

Germinal matrix

Head of caudate
nucleus

Cavum septi pellucidi

Anterior horn of
lateral ventricle

Lamina of septum
pellucidum

Putamen

External capsule

Claustrum

Anterior commissure

Substantia innominata

Globus pallidus

Anterior perforated
substance

Optic chiasm

Infundibulum

Amygdala

Uncus

Middle cerebral artery

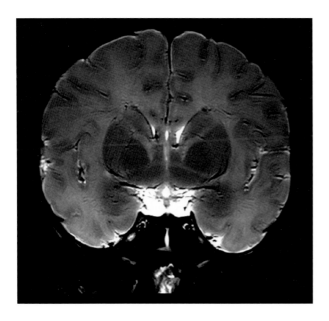

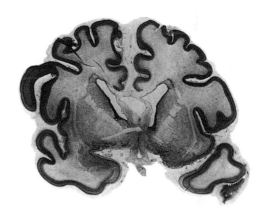

36–37 WEEKS GESTATIONAL AGE, CORONAL SECTION

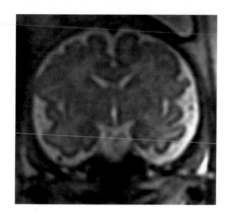

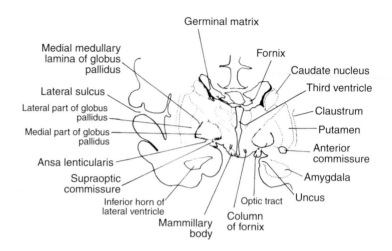

Germinal matrix

Medial medullary
lamina of globus
pallidus

Fornix

Caudate nucleus

Lateral sulcus

Third ventricle

Lateral part of globus
pallidus

Claustrum

Medial part of globus
pallidus

Putamen

Ansa lenticularis

Anterior
commissure

Supraoptic
commissure

Amygdala

Inferior horn of
lateral ventricle

Optic tract

Uncus

Mammillary
body

Column
of fornix

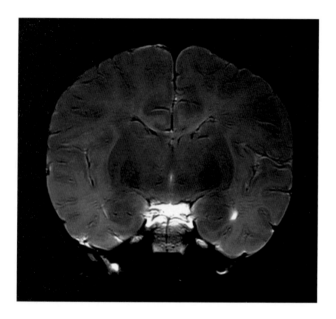

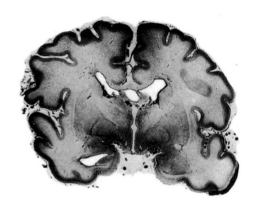

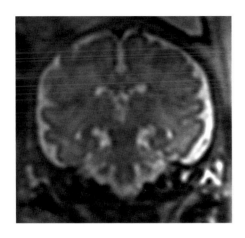

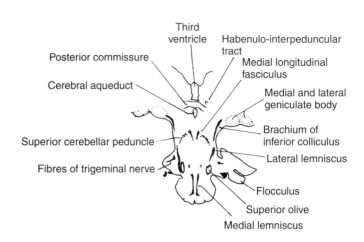

Third
ventricle

Posterior commissure

Habenulo-interpeduncular
tract

Medial longitudinal
fasciculus

Cerebral aqueduct

Medial and lateral
geniculate body

Superior cerebellar peduncle

Brachium of
inferior colliculus

Lateral lemniscus

Fibres of trigeminal nerve

Flocculus

Superior olive

Medial lemniscus

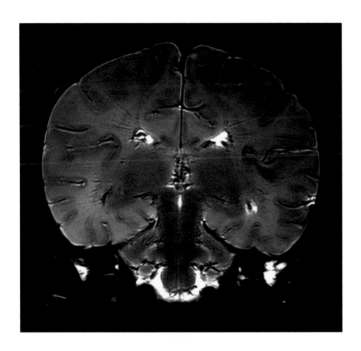

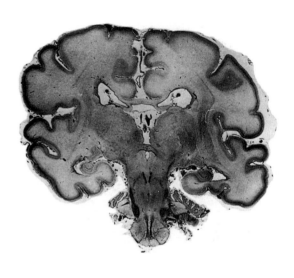

36–37 WEEKS GESTATIONAL AGE, CORONAL SECTION

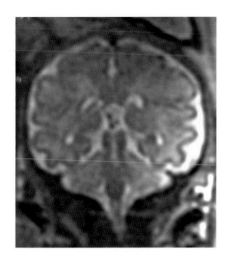

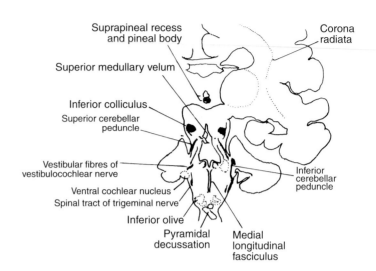

Suprapineal recess and pineal body

Corona radiata

Superior medullary velum

Inferior colliculus

Superior cerebellar peduncle

Vestibular fibres of vestibulocochlear nerve

Ventral cochlear nucleus

Spinal tract of trigeminal nerve

Inferior olive

Pyramidal decussation

Inferior cerebellar peduncle

Medial longitudinal fasciculus

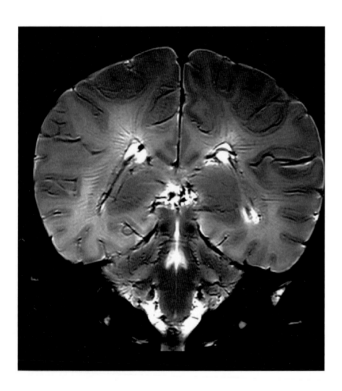

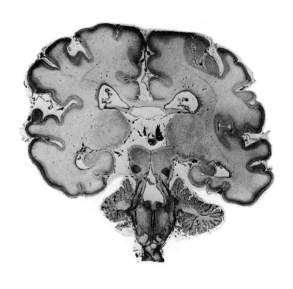

36–37 WEEKS GESTATIONAL AGE, CORONAL SECTION

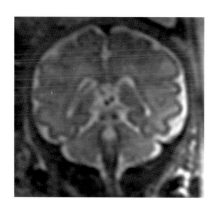

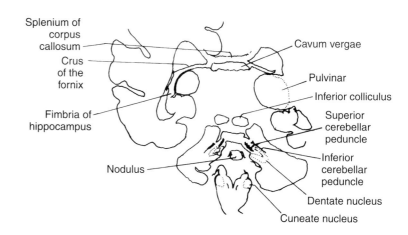

Splenium of corpus callosum

Crus of the fornix

Fimbria of hippocampus

Nodulus

Cavum vergae

Pulvinar

Inferior colliculus

Superior cerebellar peduncle

Inferior cerebellar peduncle

Dentate nucleus

Cuneate nucleus

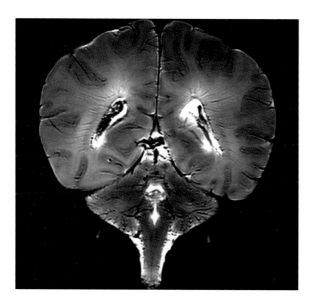

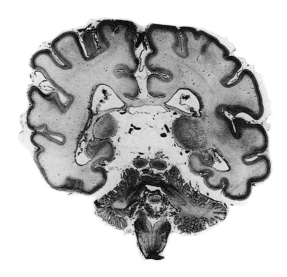

36–37 WEEKS GESTATIONAL AGE, CORONAL SECTION

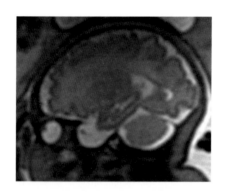

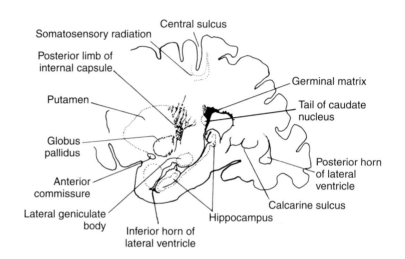

Somatosensory radiation

Central sulcus

Posterior limb of
internal capsule

Germinal matrix

Putamen

Tail of caudate
nucleus

Globus
pallidus

Posterior horn
of lateral
ventricle

Anterior
commissure

Calcarine sulcus

Lateral geniculate
body

Hippocampus

Inferior horn of
lateral ventricle

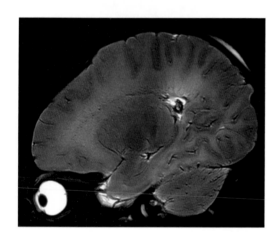

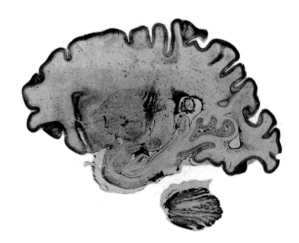

36–37 WEEKS GESTATIONAL AGE, SAGITTAL SECTION

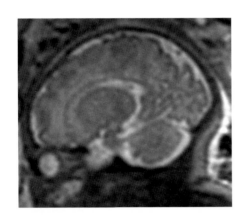

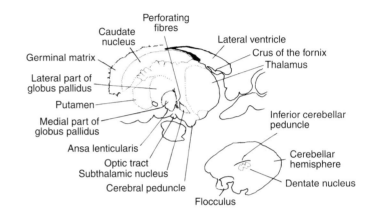

Perforating
fibres

Caudate
nucleus

Lateral ventricle

Germinal matrix

Crus of the fornix

Thalamus

Lateral part of
globus pallidus

Putamen

Medial part of
globus pallidus

Inferior cerebellar
peduncle

Ansa lenticularis

Cerebellar
hemisphere

Optic tract
Subthalamic nucleus

Dentate nucleus

Cerebral peduncle

Flocculus

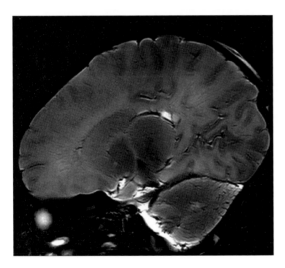

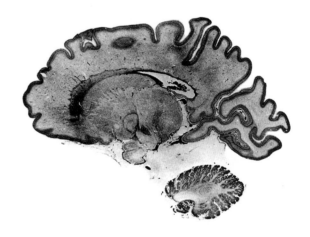

36–37 WEEKS GESTATIONAL AGE, SAGITTAL SECTION

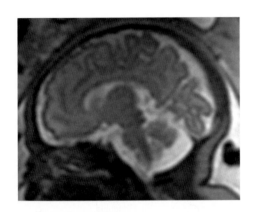

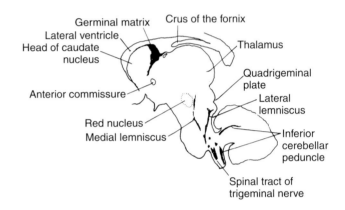

Germinal matrix — Crus of the fornix
Lateral ventricle —
Head of caudate — — Thalamus
nucleus
Anterior commissure — — Quadrigeminal
plate
— Lateral
lemniscus
Red nucleus — — Inferior
Medial lemniscus — cerebellar
peduncle
Spinal tract of
trigeminal nerve

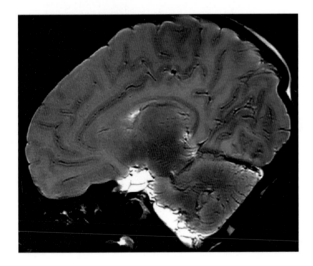

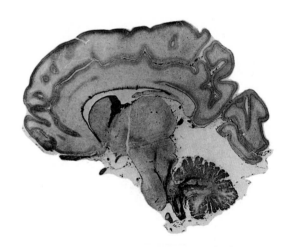

36–37 WEEKS GESTATIONAL AGE, SAGITTAL SECTION

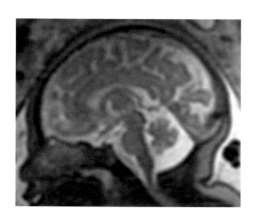

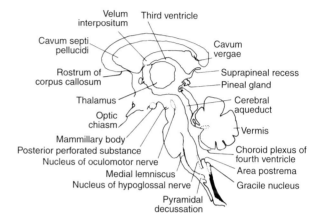

Velum interpositum

Third ventricle

Cavum septi pellucidi

Cavum vergae

Rostrum of corpus callosum

Suprapineal recess

Pineal gland

Thalamus

Cerebral aqueduct

Optic chiasm

Vermis

Mammillary body

Posterior perforated substance

Nucleus of oculomotor nerve

Choroid plexus of fourth ventricle

Area postrema

Medial lemniscus

Nucleus of hypoglossal nerve

Gracile nucleus

Pyramidal decussation

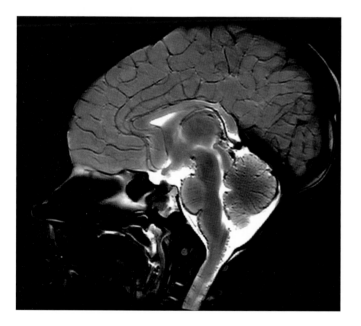

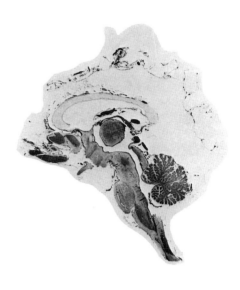

36–37 WEEKS GESTATIONAL AGE, SAGITTAL SECTION

SECTIONAL ANATOMY OF THE POSTNATAL BRAIN

This section discusses the normal magnetic resonance (MR) imaging appearance of the brains of children after term delivery up to the age of 18 months. We illustrate this topic with anatomically matched T1- and T2-weighted images and the equivalent line diagrams taken from the 40-week fetus in the Larroche atlas. The most obvious macroscopic changes that occur at this time relate to the normal, sequential changes in the degree of myelination of the brain structures. At its simplest level, MR images can be thought of as maps of body water and fat, and the changing proportions of water and lipid in brain resulting from myelination are well seen on MR images. Several groups have published data on the normal milestones of myelination and have shown how that knowledge can be used in the early detection of diseases characterized by abnormal amounts or forms of myelination.[1,2]

In the light of several years of teaching trainee radiologists, two significant, recurring misconceptions about brain myelination warrant further discussion. First, most newcomers to the field believe that no myelin at all is present in the brain of the term neonate, but this is not correct. Second, most newcomers do not appreciate that the deep brain nuclei or deep "gray matter" regions of the mature brain such as the putamen and thalamus, contain a relatively high proportion of myelin as well as cell bodies. The myelin is mainly located on projectional axons and interneurons. As a result, gray matter regions change their MR signal intensities during prenatal and postnatal life because of accumulation of myelin in them as well as in adjacent typical "white matter" structures. The signal characteristics in the deep gray matter structures are complicated further in later childhood as iron accumulates in the basal ganglia. These changes are often first seen around the age of 8 to 9 years, with rapid accumulation in the second decade of life. The iron is stored in a form that has significant effects on T2 (particularly T2′) relaxation, which explains why structures such as the globus pallidus and substantia

nigra have low T2 signal in older children and adults but not in neonates or infants.

A good example of the competing signal changes brought about by these mechanisms is illustrated by the T2 signal of the globus pallidus and putamen at different ages. These structures provide useful comparison because they are both deep gray matter nuclei and their close anatomic proximity allows direct comparison. The two structures would be predicted to have similar signal characteristics because they have similar neuronal/glial composition. This is true for the first 30 to 32 weeks of gestation. However, myelination proceeds more rapidly in the globus pallidus when compared with the putamen (even in the posterior portion of the putamen that myelinates first). This difference usually can be seen as lower signal in the globus pallidus on T2-weighted images at 33 to 34 weeks' gestational age. As myelination proceeds in both structures, the signal differential reduces, and at 0 to 1 months post term little signal difference is seen, a characteristic that is maintained for a number of years. The accumulation of iron in brain structures is exceptionally variable by region and continues throughout life. MR techniques that can quantify the amount of iron deposition are available.[3] However, the globus pallidus accumulates iron particularly rapidly and to high concentration. A higher concentration of iron is present in the normal adult globus pallidus than in the liver. After 7 to 8 years of age, the globus pallidus usually has lower signal than the putamen on T2-weighted images, a feature that is most marked on imaging at higher field strengths (e.g., 3 T).

Macroscopic myelination before term has been studied using both fixed and appropriately stained fetal tissue and MR imaging. Good correlation between the two techniques has been observed, particularly if increased signal on T1-weighted images is used to evaluate early postnatal myelination. Evidence of supratentorial myelination is unusual in the 29- to 30-week fetus/premature baby. Consistent evidence of supratentorial myelination at any site is seen on MR imaging only at 33 to 34 weeks. High T1 signal at that stage is frequently seen in the thalamus (particularly ventrolateral) and putamen (particularly posteriorly); the lateral thalamic regions and globus pallidus may also show reduced signal on T2-weighted images. By 37 to 38 weeks, the high T1 signal intensity has increased generally in the basal ganglia and thalami, and evidence of myelination in the posterior limb of the internal capsule and the corona radiata close to the ventricles is seen. Most of those regions also return low signal on T2-weighted images around that maturity (Figure 3-1).

Myelination is more advanced in the infratentorial brain structures. By 33 to 34 weeks, prominent signal changes consistent with myelination on both T1 and T2 sequences are seen in most of the dorsal pons and medulla and in the deep cerebellar white matter. High-resolution studies show myelination within the inferior colliculus and medial lemniscus. By 37 to 38 weeks, prominent myelination usually is seen in the superior cerebellar peduncle, most of the midbrain, and the cerebellar white matter. A 38-week example is shown in Figure 3-2.

There is close correlation between the regions of the brain injured close to term by profound, hypoxic ischemic injury and the regions of the brain that are actively myelinating. For example, a typical textbook description of a close-to-term profound ischemic injury includes involvement of the lateral thalamus, posterior putamen, white matter of the paracentral lobule, and optic radiations (Figure 3-3).[1,2] These are precisely the regions that show

low T2 signal due to myelin formation in the 38-week fetus. It has been postulated that there is a selective vulnerability for regions of the brain that are metabolically active in the face of hypoxia/ischemia. In the brain of the term neonate this does not necessarily imply neuronal activity; it is much more likely that myelination is the most energy-dependent process. This goes a significant way towards explaining the pattern of injuries seen on neuroimaging and this has helped to explain why some less-well described regions of the brain, such as the anterior lobule of the cerebellar vermis[3,4] and the subthalamic nucleus,[5] are also involved in the process. Our interest in the involvement of the subthalamic nucleus in cases of profound hypoxic ischemic injury has come about because of the central role of that structure in suppressing unwanted movements acting in parallel to volitional movement. It is no surprise to find that the subthalamic nucleus myelinates close to term (Figure 3-4).

Detailed descriptions of myelination can be reviewed in other more specific texts,[1] but using the physical explanations outlined earlier in the introduction we can produce a list of key features that may be useful in clinical practice.

- Mature myelin has high signal on T1-weighted images (compared to gray matter).
- Mature myelin has low signal on T2-weighted images (compared to gray matter).
- T1-weighted images should show the expected high signal in all white matter regions by the age of 8 months (i.e., myelination is virtually adult pattern at 8 months).

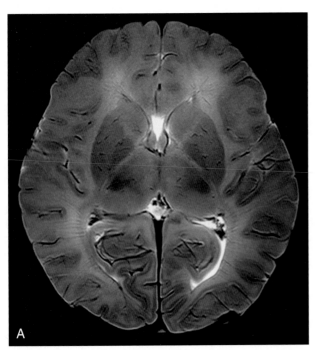
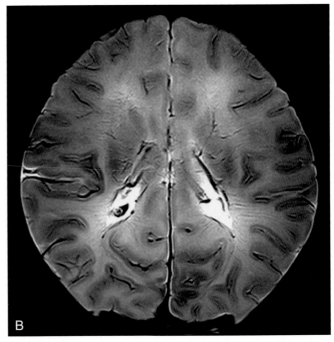

Figure 3-1   T2-weighted images of the supratentorial brain from a postmortem magnetic resonance imaging study of a 38-week fetus with normal brain anatomy performed at 3 T. Note the low-signal regions that are most prominent within the lateral thalamus, globus pallidus, putamen **(A)**, and central corona radiata **(B)**.

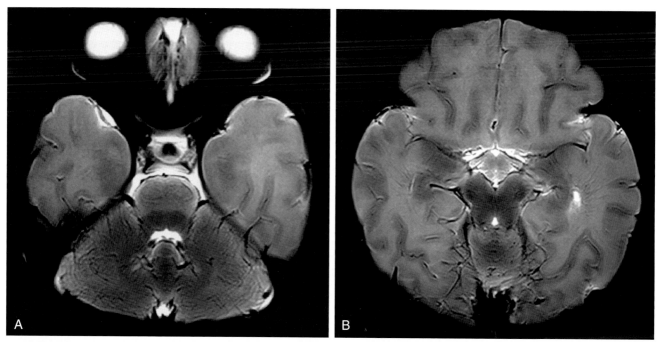

Figure 3-2   T2-weighted images of the infratentorial brain from a postmortem magnetic resonance imaging study of a 38-week fetus with normal brain anatomy image performed at 3 T. Note the low-signal regions that are most prominent within the dorsal brainstem, superior cerebellar peduncle **(A)**, and anterior lobule of the cerebellar vermis **(B)**.

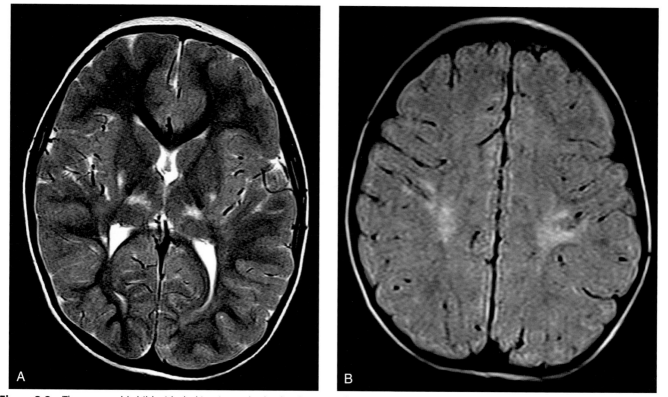

Figure 3-3   Three-year-old child with dyskinetic cerebral palsy due to profound hypoxic ischemic injury at birth (38 weeks' gestation). **A,** Axial T2-weighted image at the level of the basal ganglia/thalami showing gliosis (high signal) in the posterior putamen and ventral lateral thalamic nuclei. **B,** Axial fluid attenuation inversion recovery (FLAIR) image toward the vertex showing gliosis in the paracentral white matter. The affected regions were actively myelinating at the time of the injury, which may contribute to the selective vulnerability of those structures.

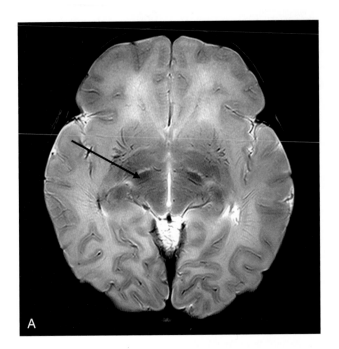
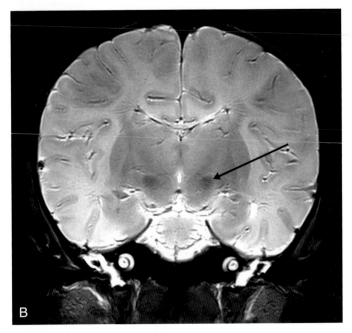
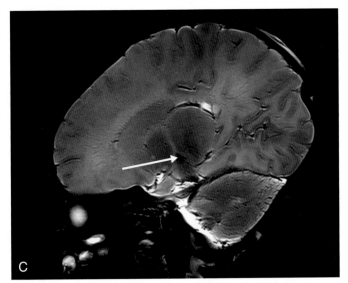

Figure 3-4   T2-weighted postmortem magnetic resonance images of a 38-week fetus at 3 T with no structural brain abnormality showing myelination in the subthalamic nucleus *(arrow)* in the axial **(A)**, coronal **(B)**, and parasagittal **(C)** planes.

TABLE 3-1

Checklist for Normal Myelination: Structures That Should Appear Myelinated by the Specified Age

T1	T2
0–1 Month	
Dorsal brainstem	Dorsal brainstem
Inferior and middle cerebellar peduncles	Inferior cerebellar peduncles
Superior cerebellar peduncles and decussation	Superior cerebellar peduncles and decussation
Ventral lateral thalamus	Ventral lateral thalamus
Posterior putamen	Posterior putamen
White matter of pre and postcentral gyri	White matter of pre- and postcentral gyri
Optic tracts	Optic tracts
Posterior limb of internal capsule	Posterior limb of internal capsule (patchy and limited to posterior region)
Central portion of centrum semiovale	
Optic radiations	
3–4 Months	
All of the above	All of the above
All of the cerebellum	Middle cerebellar peduncle
Ventral brainstem	Ventral brainstem
Calcarine fissure white matter	Calcarine fissure white matter
All subcortical motor pathways	Optic radiations
Anterior limb of internal capsule	
Splenium of corpus callosum	
6 Months	
All but subcortical white matter	Centrum semiovale
	All of posterior limb of internal capsule
	Patchy changes in anterior limb of internal capsule
	Splenium of corpus callosum
	Patchy changes in genu of corpus callosum
9 Months	
Adult pattern	Genu of corpus callosum
	Centrum semiovale
12 Months	
Adult pattern	All of internal capsule
	All of corpus callosum
	Paracentral and optic radiations/paracalcarine white matter
18 Months	
Adult pattern	Adult pattern except most peripheral cortical white matter
	Peritrigonal white matter can return high signal until the fourth decade (terminal myelination zones)

- T2-weighted images should show the expected low signal in all white matter regions by the age of 24 months (except peritrigonal "terminal myelination" zones).
- Myelination proceeds in an anatomically predictable fashion in normal children, a process that must be understood by anyone reporting MR examinations in children at this age. See Table 3-1.

- T1-weighted images are best for assessing myelination before the age of 8 months (except brainstem and cerebellum) and T2-weighted images thereafter, although both should be acquired and compared.

The remainder of this chapter demonstrates T1- and T2-weighted images from birth to 18 months in order to show the evolution of myelination.

REFERENCES

1. Barkovich AJ: Pediatric Neuroimaging, 4th ed. Philadelphia, Lippincott Williams & Wilkins, 2005.
2. van der Knapp M, Valk J: Magnetic Resonance of Myelin, Myelination and Myelin Disorders, 2nd ed. Berlin, Springer, 1995.
3. Sargent MA, Poskitt KJ, Roland EH, Hill A, Hendson G: Cerebellar vermian atrophy after neonatal hypoxic ischemic encephalopathy. Am J Neuroradiol 25:1008–1015, 2004.
4. Connolly DJA, Widjaja E, Griffiths PD: Involvement of the anterior lobe of the cerebellar vermis in perinatal profound hypoxia. Am J Neuroradiol 28:16–19, 2007.

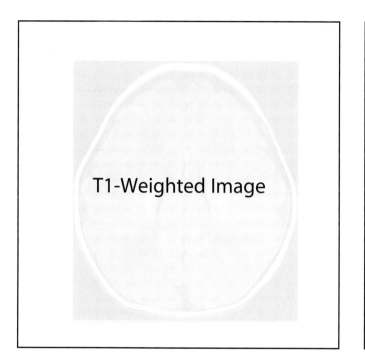

T1-Weighted Image

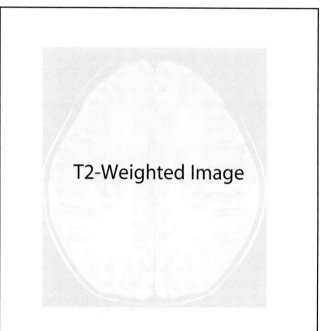

T2-Weighted Image

Line Diagram

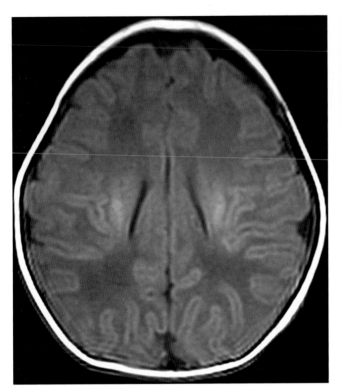
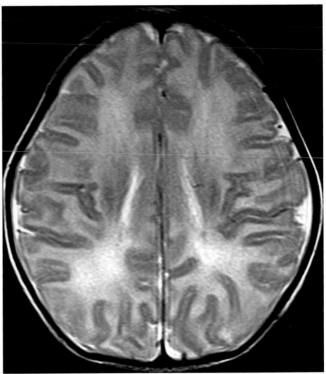

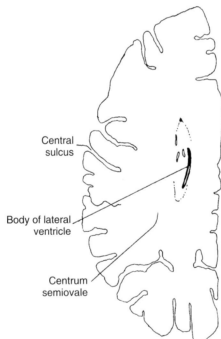

Central
sulcus

Body of lateral
ventricle

Centrum
semiovale

POSTNATAL MR 0–1 MONTH, AXIAL

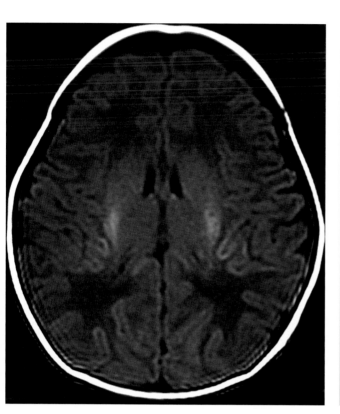
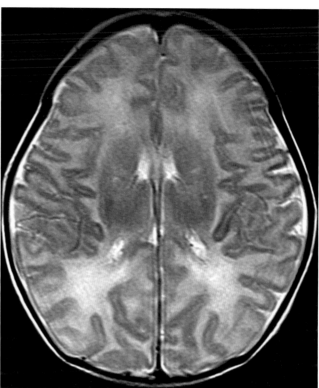

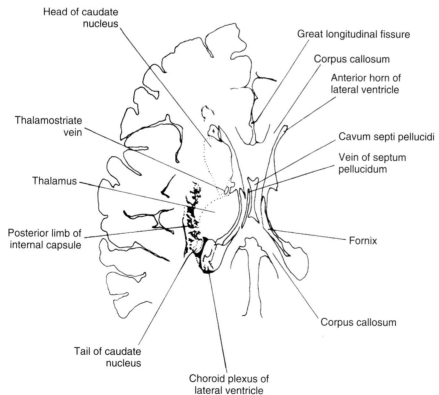

Head of caudate nucleus

Great longitudinal fissure

Corpus callosum

Anterior horn of lateral ventricle

Thalamostriate vein

Cavum septi pellucidi

Vein of septum pellucidum

Thalamus

Posterior limb of internal capsule

Fornix

Corpus callosum

Tail of caudate nucleus

Choroid plexus of lateral ventricle

POSTNATAL MR 0–1 MONTH, AXIAL

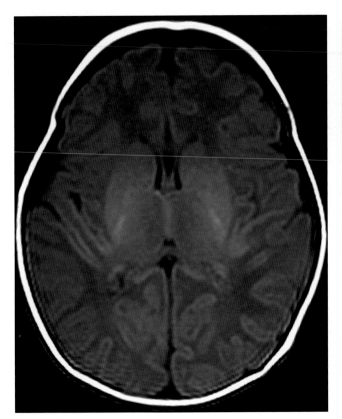
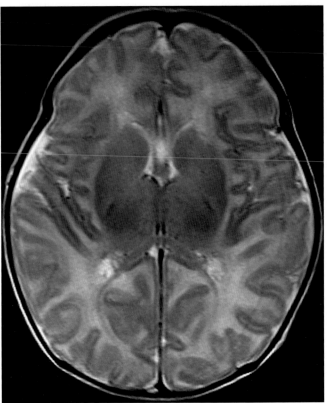

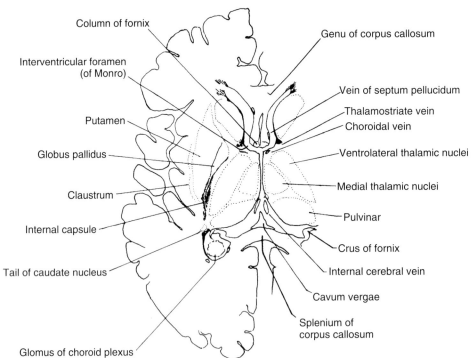

Column of fornix

Interventricular foramen
(of Monro)

Putamen

Globus pallidus

Claustrum

Internal capsule

Tail of caudate nucleus

Glomus of choroid plexus

Genu of corpus callosum

Vein of septum pellucidum

Thalamostriate vein

Choroidal vein

Ventrolateral thalamic nuclei

Medial thalamic nuclei

Pulvinar

Crus of fornix

Internal cerebral vein

Cavum vergae

Splenium of
corpus callosum

POSTNATAL MR 0–1 MONTH, AXIAL

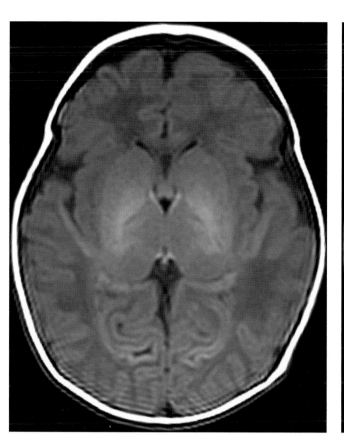
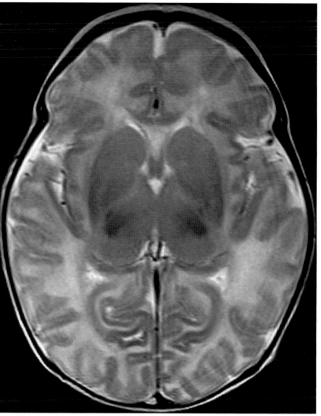

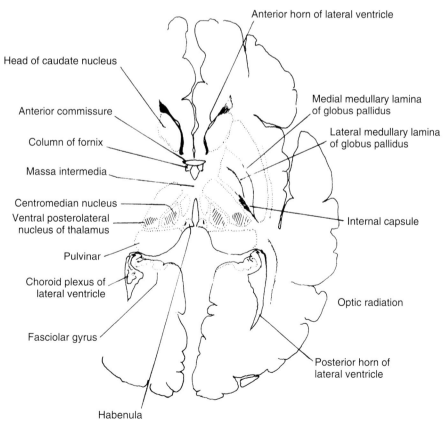

Anterior horn of lateral ventricle

Head of caudate nucleus

Anterior commissure

Column of fornix

Massa intermedia

Centromedian nucleus

Ventral posterolateral nucleus of thalamus

Pulvinar

Choroid plexus of lateral ventricle

Fasciolar gyrus

Habenula

Medial medullary lamina of globus pallidus

Lateral medullary lamina of globus pallidus

Internal capsule

Optic radiation

Posterior horn of lateral ventricle

POSTNATAL MR 0–1 MONTH, AXIAL

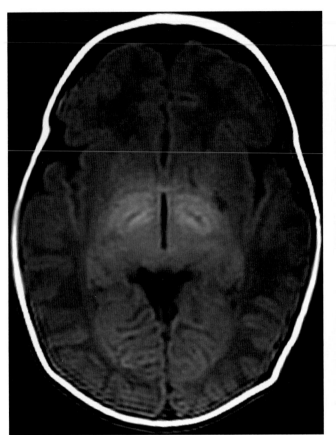
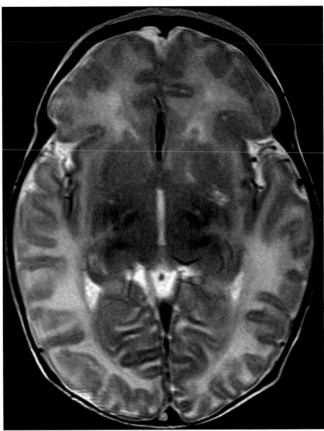

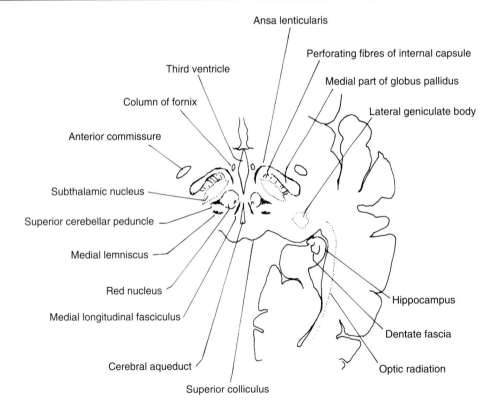

Ansa lenticularis

Perforating fibres of internal capsule

Third ventricle

Medial part of globus pallidus

Column of fornix

Lateral geniculate body

Anterior commissure

Subthalamic nucleus

Superior cerebellar peduncle

Medial lemniscus

Red nucleus

Hippocampus

Medial longitudinal fasciculus

Dentate fascia

Cerebral aqueduct

Optic radiation

Superior colliculus

POSTNATAL MR 0–1 MONTH, AXIAL

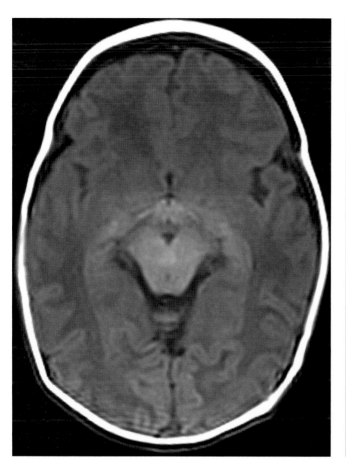
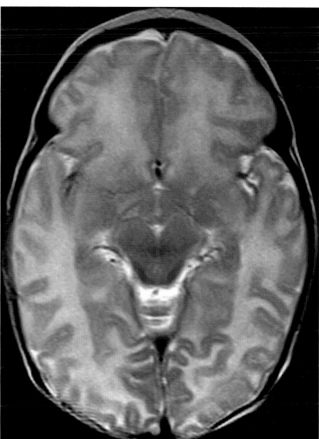

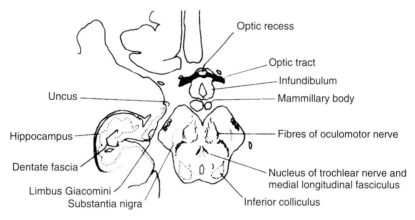

Optic recess

Optic tract

Infundibulum

Uncus

Mammillary body

Hippocampus

Fibres of oculomotor nerve

Dentate fascia

Nucleus of trochlear nerve and medial longitudinal fasciculus

Limbus Giacomini

Substantia nigra

Inferior colliculus

POSTNATAL MR 0–1 MONTH, AXIAL

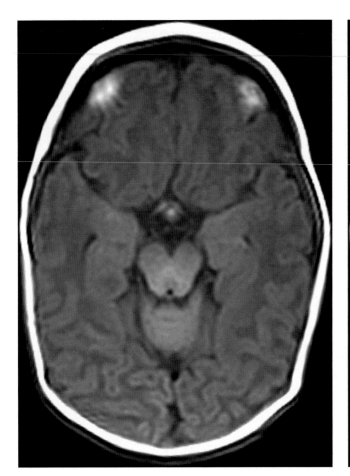
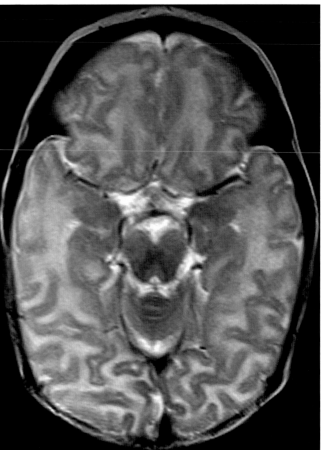

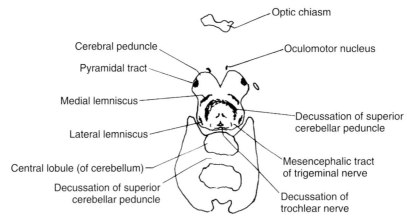

Optic chiasm

Cerebral peduncle

Oculomotor nucleus

Pyramidal tract

Medial lemniscus

Decussation of superior
cerebellar peduncle

Lateral lemniscus

Mesencephalic tract
of trigeminal nerve

Central lobule (of cerebellum)

Decussation of superior
cerebellar peduncle

Decussation of
trochlear nerve

POSTNATAL MR 0–1 MONTH, AXIAL

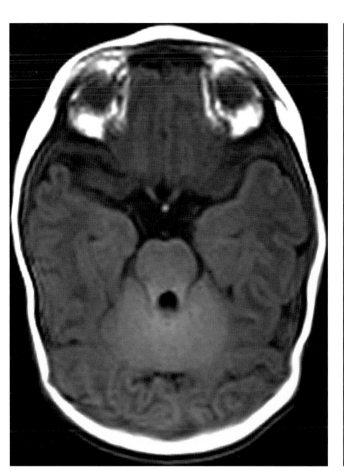
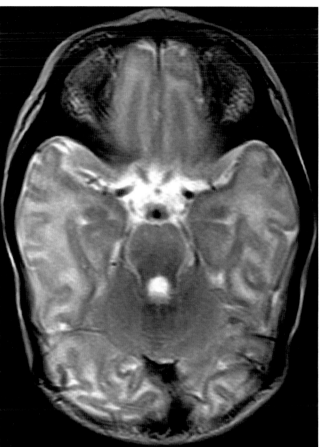

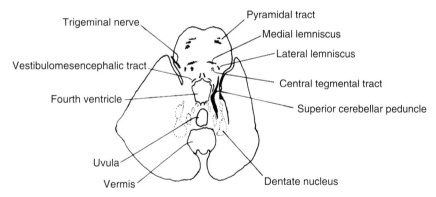

Trigeminal nerve

Pyramidal tract

Medial lemniscus

Lateral lemniscus

Vestibulomesencephalic tract

Central tegmental tract

Fourth ventricle

Superior cerebellar peduncle

Uvula

Vermis

Dentate nucleus

POSTNATAL MR 0–1 MONTH, AXIAL

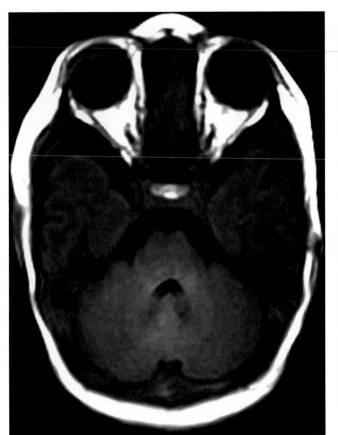
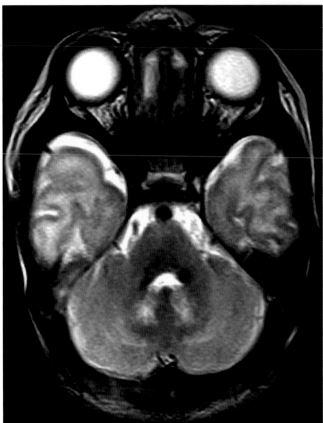

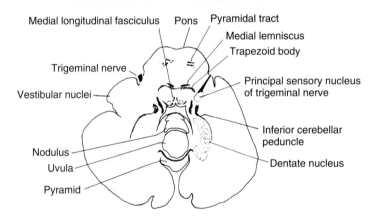

Medial longitudinal fasciculus — Pons — Pyramidal tract

Medial lemniscus

Trapezoid body

Trigeminal nerve

Principal sensory nucleus
of trigeminal nerve

Vestibular nuclei

Inferior cerebellar
peduncle

Nodulus

Uvula

Dentate nucleus

Pyramid

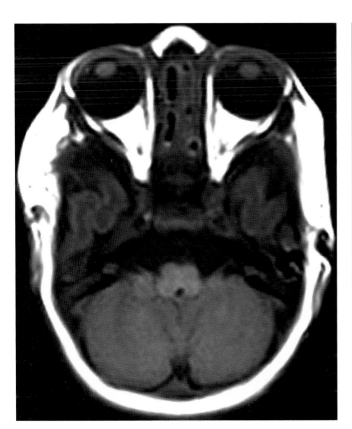
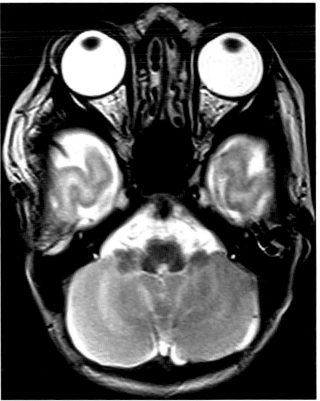

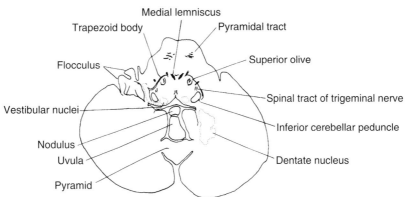

Medial lemniscus

Trapezoid body

Pyramidal tract

Flocculus

Superior olive

Spinal tract of trigeminal nerve

Vestibular nuclei

Inferior cerebellar peduncle

Nodulus

Uvula

Dentate nucleus

Pyramid

POSTNATAL MR 0–1 MONTH, AXIAL

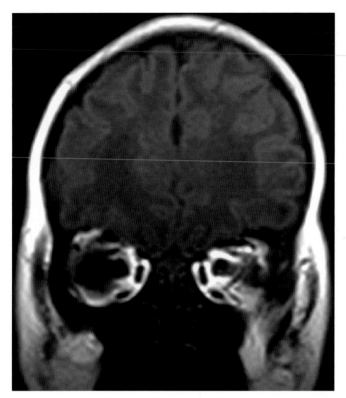
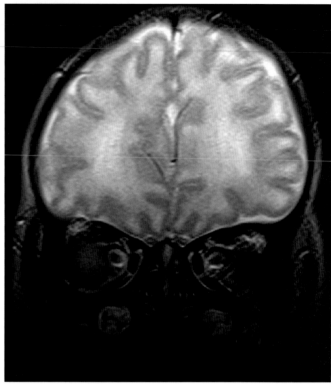

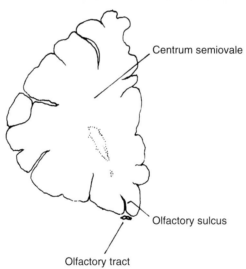

Centrum semiovale

Olfactory sulcus

Olfactory tract

POSTNATAL MR 0–1 MONTH, CORONAL

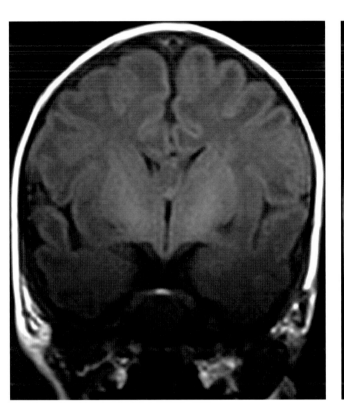
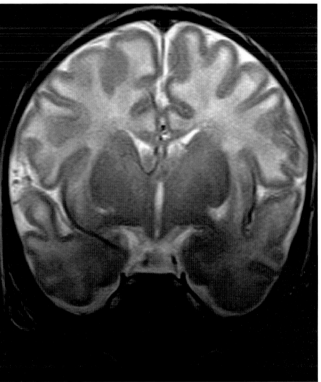

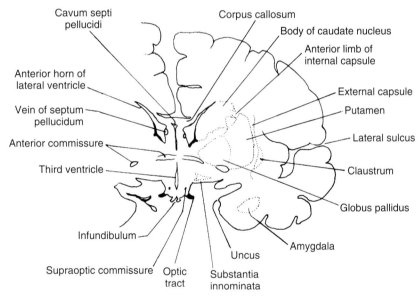

Cavum septi pellucidi

Anterior horn of lateral ventricle

Vein of septum pellucidum

Anterior commissure

Third ventricle

Infundibulum

Supraoptic commissure

Optic tract

Substantia innominata

Uncus

Amygdala

Globus pallidus

Claustrum

Lateral sulcus

Putamen

External capsule

Anterior limb of internal capsule

Body of caudate nucleus

Corpus callosum

POSTNATAL MR 0–1 MONTH, CORONAL

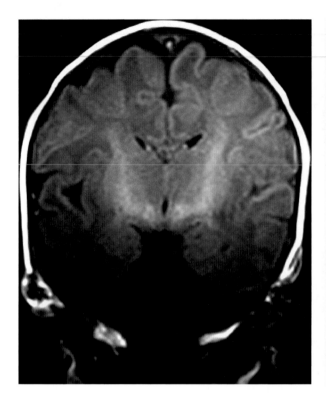
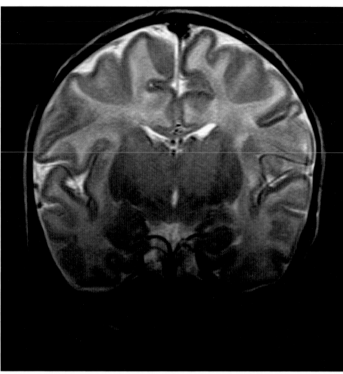

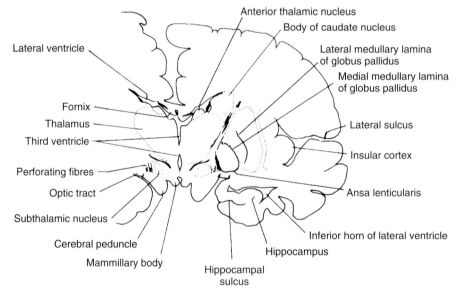

Anterior thalamic nucleus

Body of caudate nucleus

Lateral medullary lamina of globus pallidus

Medial medullary lamina of globus pallidus

Lateral ventricle

Lateral sulcus

Fornix

Insular cortex

Thalamus

Third ventricle

Perforating fibres

Ansa lenticularis

Optic tract

Subthalamic nucleus

Cerebral peduncle

Inferior horn of lateral ventricle

Hippocampus

Mammillary body

Hippocampal sulcus

POSTNATAL MR 0–1 MONTH, CORONAL

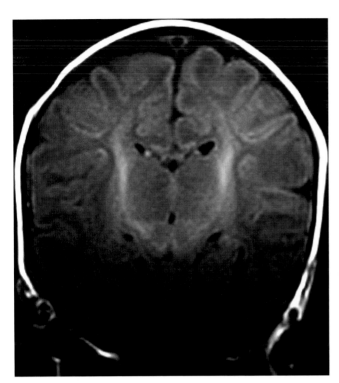
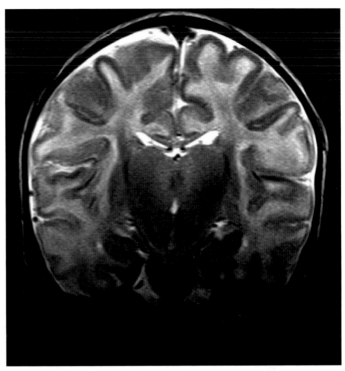

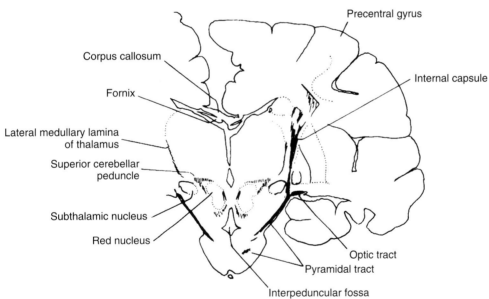

POSTNATAL MR 0-1 MONTH, CORONAL

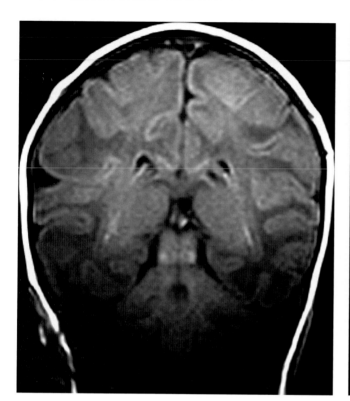
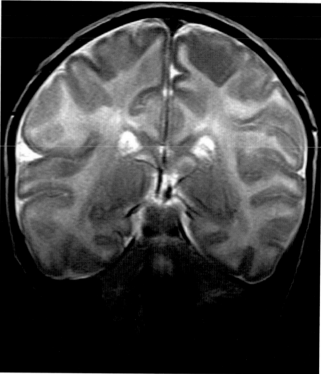

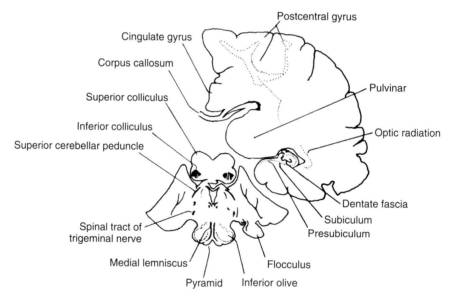

POSTNATAL MR 0–1 MONTH, CORONAL

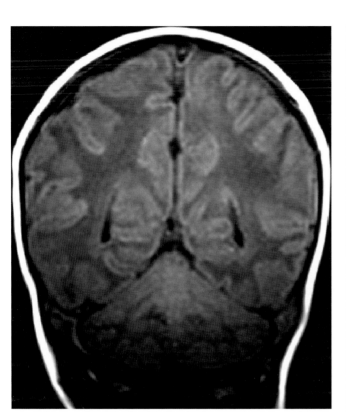
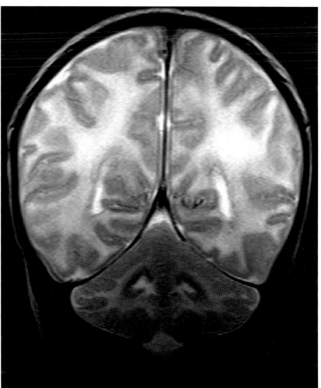

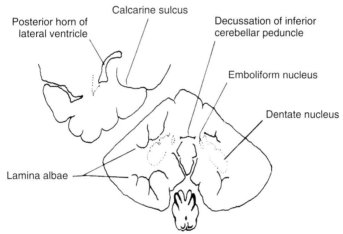

Posterior horn of lateral ventricle

Calcarine sulcus

Decussation of inferior cerebellar peduncle

Emboliform nucleus

Dentate nucleus

Lamina albae

POSTNATAL MR 0–1 MONTH, SAGITTAL

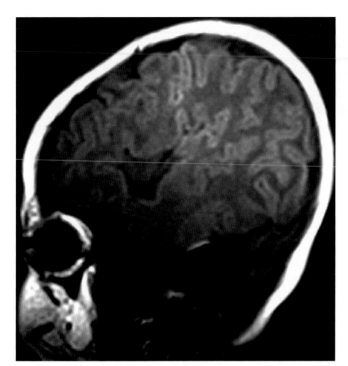
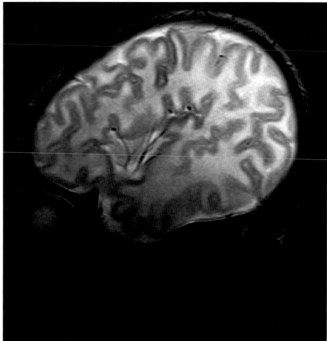

Lateral sulcus

Superior temporal sulcus

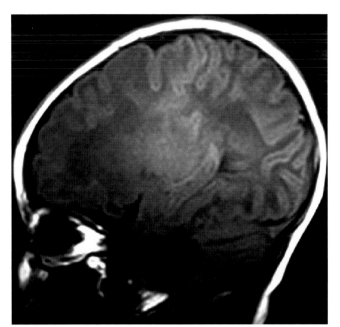
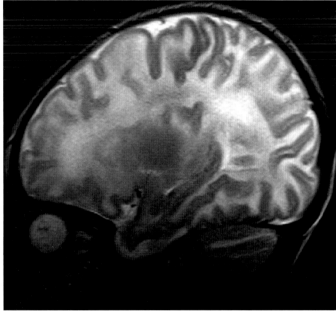

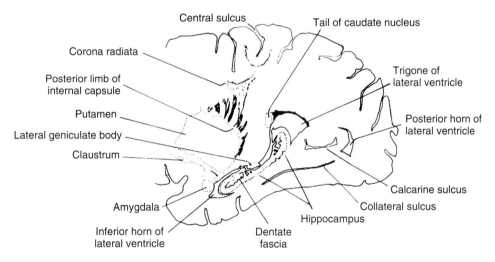

Central sulcus

Tail of caudate nucleus

Corona radiata

Trigone of
lateral ventricle

Posterior limb of
internal capsule

Putamen

Posterior horn of
lateral ventricle

Lateral geniculate body

Claustrum

Calcarine sulcus

Amygdala

Collateral sulcus

Hippocampus

Inferior horn of
lateral ventricle

Dentate
fascia

POSTNATAL MR 0–1 MONTH, SAGITTAL

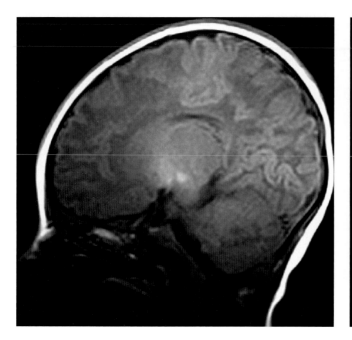
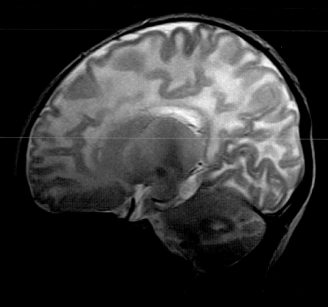

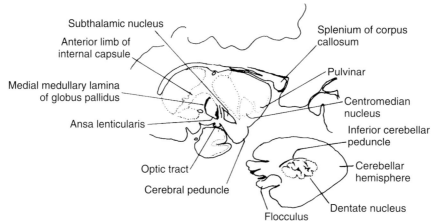

Subthalamic nucleus

Anterior limb of
internal capsule

Medial medullary lamina
of globus pallidus

Ansa lenticularis

Optic tract

Cerebral peduncle

Splenium of corpus
callosum

Pulvinar

Centromedian
nucleus

Inferior cerebellar
peduncle

Cerebellar
hemisphere

Dentate nucleus

Flocculus

POSTNATAL MR 0–1 MONTH, SAGITTAL

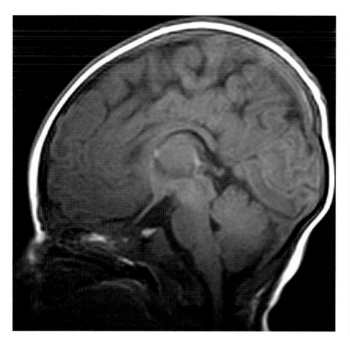
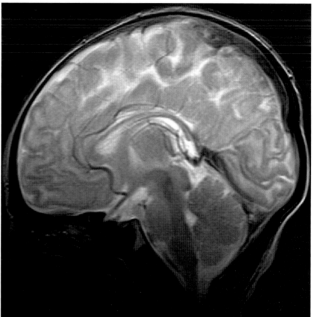

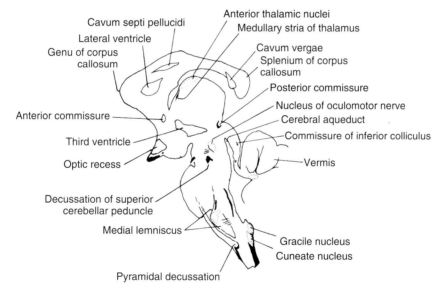

Cavum septi pellucidi

Anterior thalamic nuclei
Medullary stria of thalamus

Lateral ventricle

Genu of corpus
callosum

Cavum vergae
Splenium of corpus
callosum

Posterior commissure

Anterior commissure

Nucleus of oculomotor nerve
Cerebral aqueduct

Third ventricle

Commissure of inferior colliculus

Optic recess

Vermis

Decussation of superior
cerebellar peduncle

Medial lemniscus

Gracile nucleus
Cuneate nucleus

Pyramidal decussation

POSTNATAL MR 0–1 MONTH, SAGITTAL

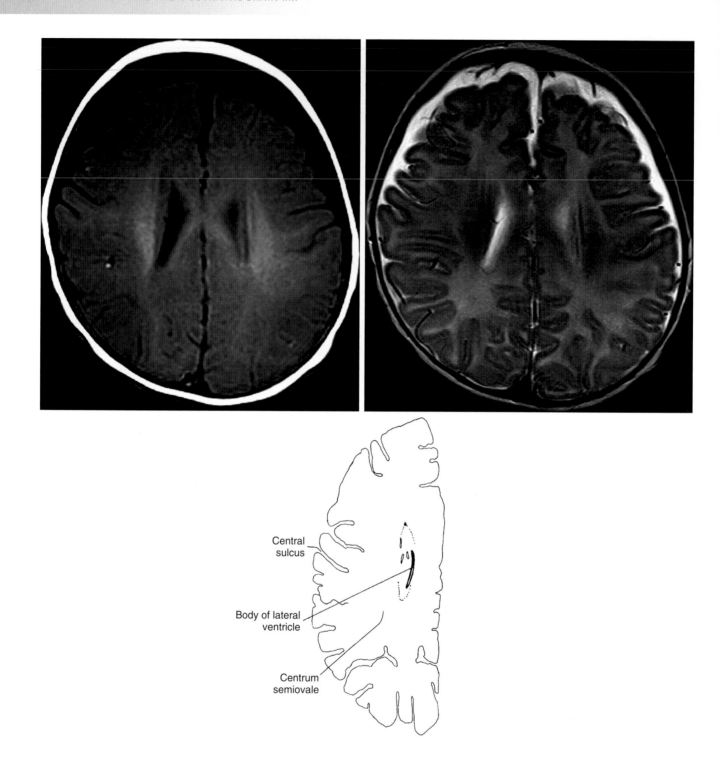

Central
sulcus

Body of lateral
ventricle

Centrum
semiovale

POSTNATAL MR 3–4 MONTHS, AXIAL

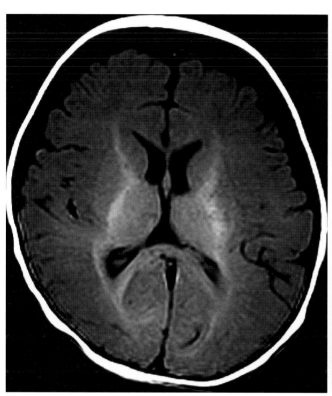
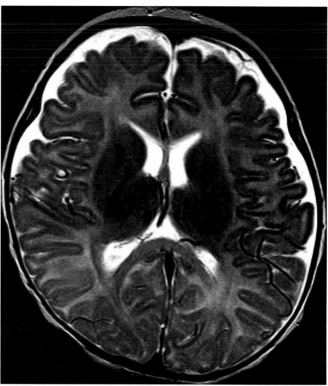
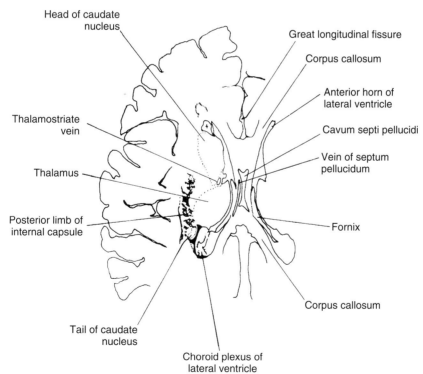

Head of caudate nucleus

Great longitudinal fissure

Corpus callosum

Anterior horn of lateral ventricle

Thalamostriate vein

Cavum septi pellucidi

Vein of septum pellucidum

Thalamus

Posterior limb of internal capsule

Fornix

Corpus callosum

Tail of caudate nucleus

Choroid plexus of lateral ventricle

POSTNATAL MR 3–4 MONTHS, AXIAL

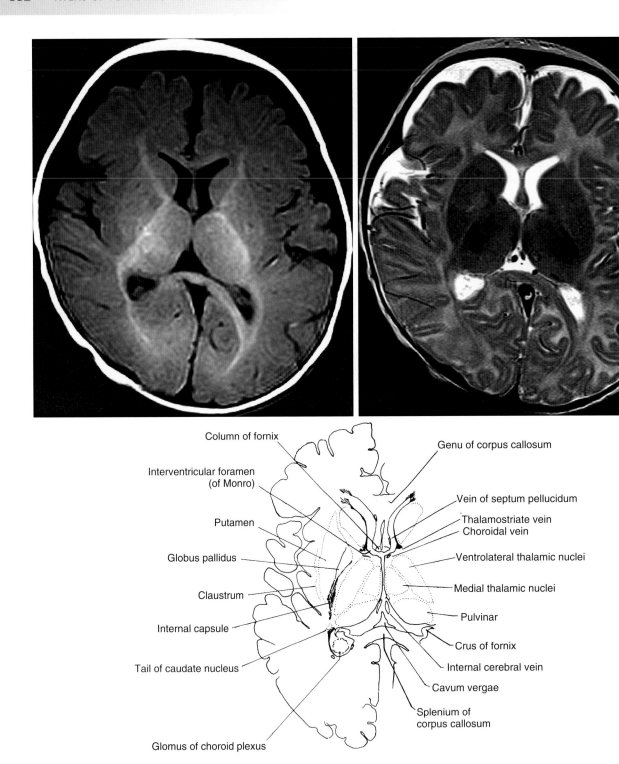

Column of fornix

Interventricular foramen
(of Monro)

Putamen

Globus pallidus

Claustrum

Internal capsule

Tail of caudate nucleus

Glomus of choroid plexus

Genu of corpus callosum

Vein of septum pellucidum

Thalamostriate vein
Choroidal vein

Ventrolateral thalamic nuclei

Medial thalamic nuclei

Pulvinar

Crus of fornix

Internal cerebral vein

Cavum vergae

Splenium of
corpus callosum

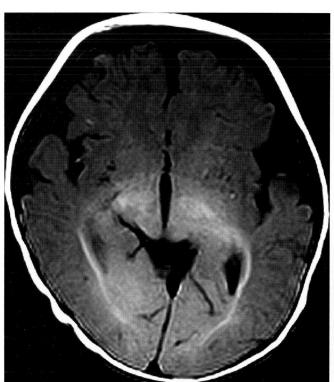
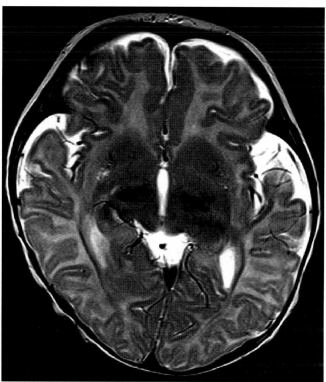

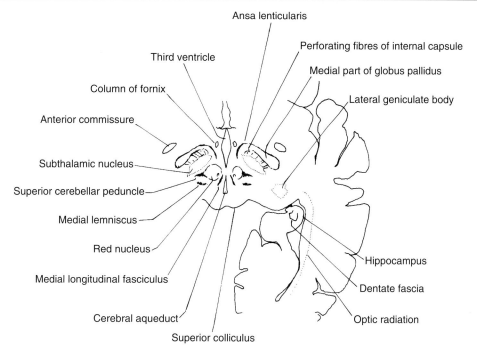

Ansa lenticularis

Perforating fibres of internal capsule

Third ventricle

Medial part of globus pallidus

Column of fornix

Lateral geniculate body

Anterior commissure

Subthalamic nucleus

Superior cerebellar peduncle

Medial lemniscus

Red nucleus

Hippocampus

Medial longitudinal fasciculus

Dentate fascia

Cerebral aqueduct

Optic radiation

Superior colliculus

POSTNATAL MR 3–4 MONTHS, AXIAL

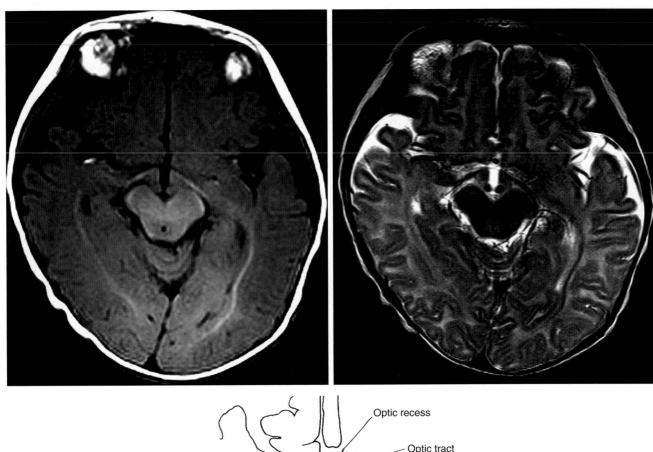

POSTNATAL MR 3–4 MONTHS, AXIAL

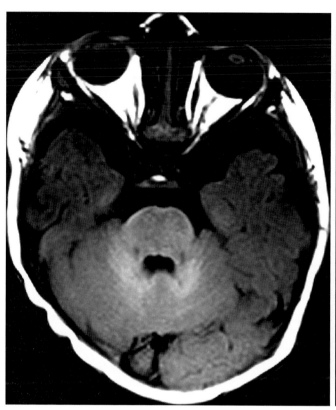
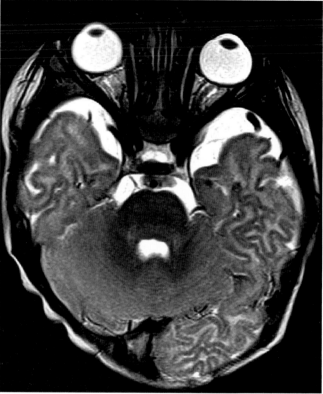

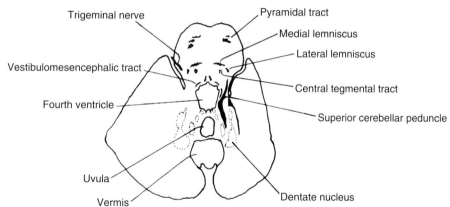

Trigeminal nerve

Pyramidal tract

Medial lemniscus

Lateral lemniscus

Vestibulomesencephalic tract

Central tegmental tract

Fourth ventricle

Superior cerebellar peduncle

Uvula

Vermis

Dentate nucleus

POSTNATAL MR 3–4 MONTHS, AXIAL

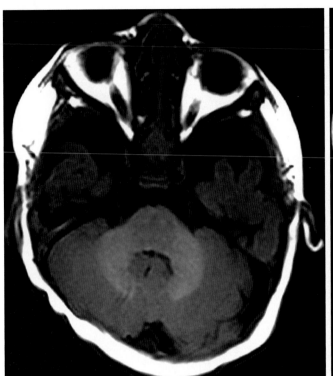
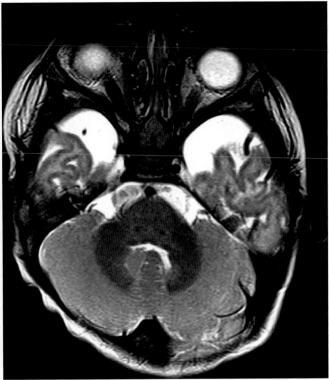

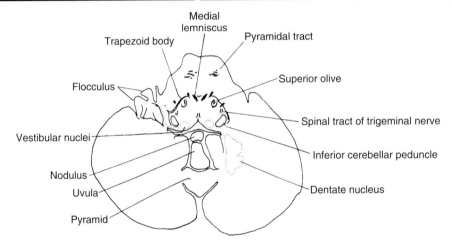

Medial lemniscus

Trapezoid body

Pyramidal tract

Flocculus

Superior olive

Spinal tract of trigeminal nerve

Vestibular nuclei

Inferior cerebellar peduncle

Nodulus

Dentate nucleus

Uvula

Pyramid

POSTNATAL MR 3–4 MONTHS, AXIAL

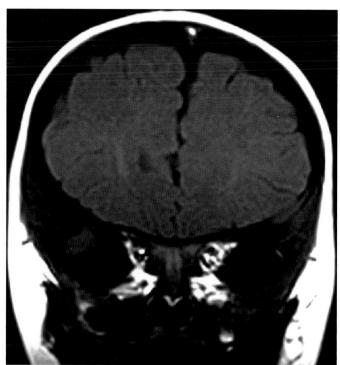
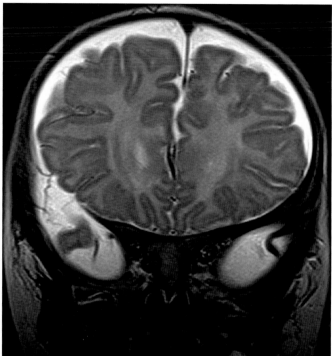

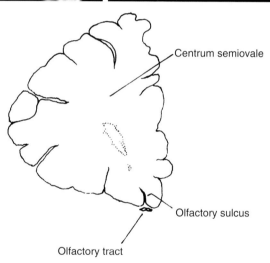

Centrum semiovale

Olfactory sulcus

Olfactory tract

POSTNATAL MR 3–4 MONTHS, AXIAL

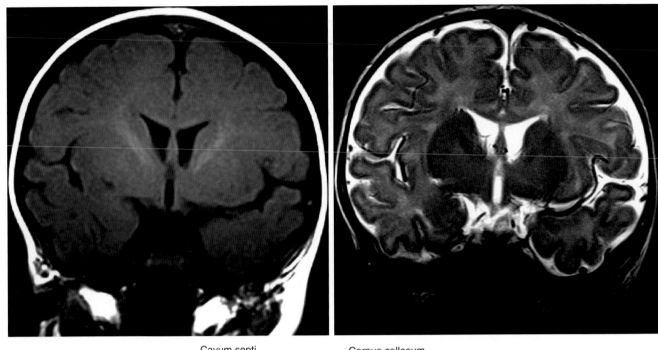

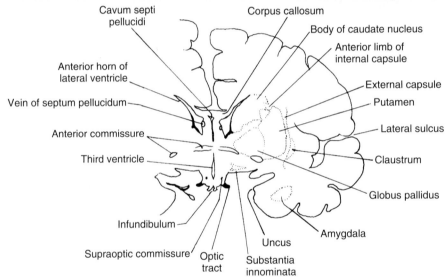

Cavum septi pellucidi

Corpus callosum

Body of caudate nucleus

Anterior limb of internal capsule

Anterior horn of lateral ventricle

External capsule

Putamen

Vein of septum pellucidum

Lateral sulcus

Anterior commissure

Claustrum

Third ventricle

Globus pallidus

Infundibulum

Amygdala

Supraoptic commissure

Optic tract

Uncus

Substantia innominata

POSTNATAL MR 3–4 MONTHS, AXIAL

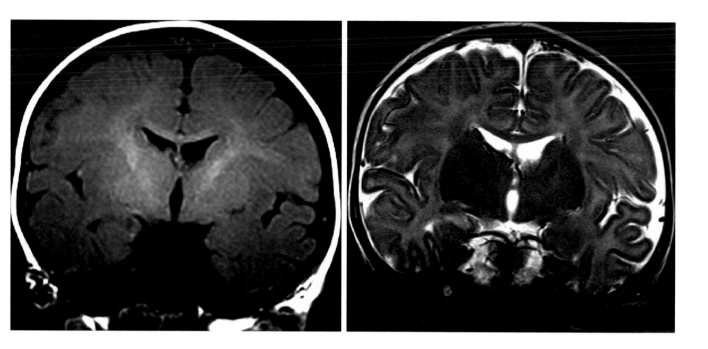

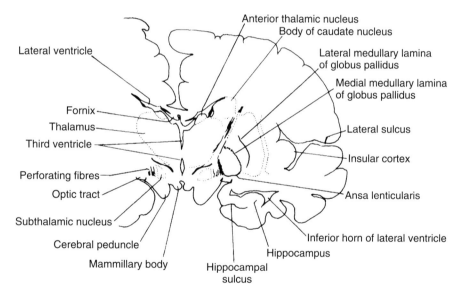

Anterior thalamic nucleus

Body of caudate nucleus

Lateral ventricle

Lateral medullary lamina of globus pallidus

Medial medullary lamina of globus pallidus

Fornix

Thalamus

Lateral sulcus

Third ventricle

Insular cortex

Perforating fibres

Optic tract

Ansa lenticularis

Subthalamic nucleus

Cerebral peduncle

Inferior horn of lateral ventricle

Hippocampus

Mammillary body

Hippocampal sulcus

POSTNATAL MR 3–4 MONTHS, AXIAL

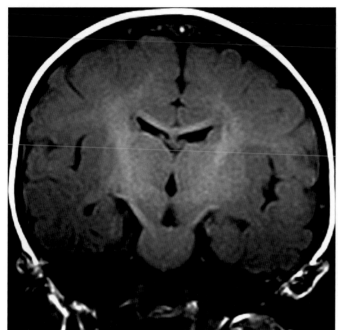
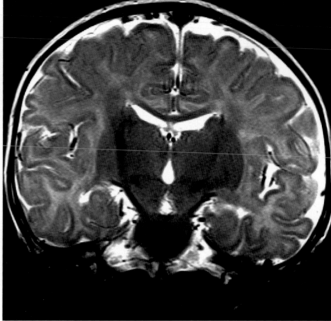

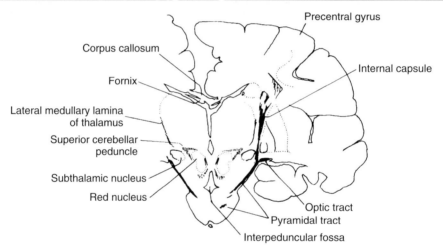

Corpus callosum

Fornix

Lateral medullary lamina
of thalamus

Superior cerebellar
peduncle

Subthalamic nucleus

Red nucleus

Precentral gyrus

Internal capsule

Optic tract

Pyramidal tract

Interpeduncular fossa

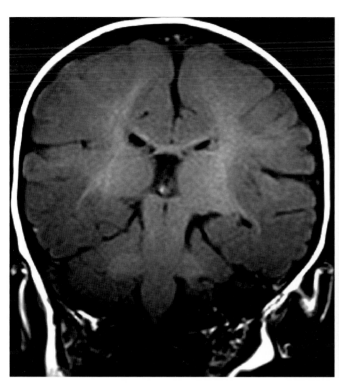
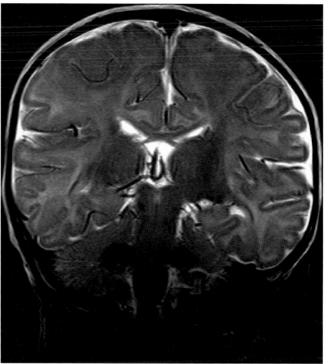

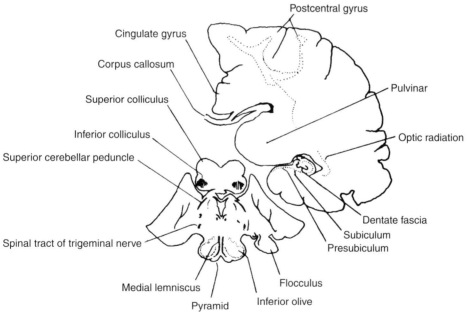

POSTNATAL MR 3–4 MONTHS, CORONAL

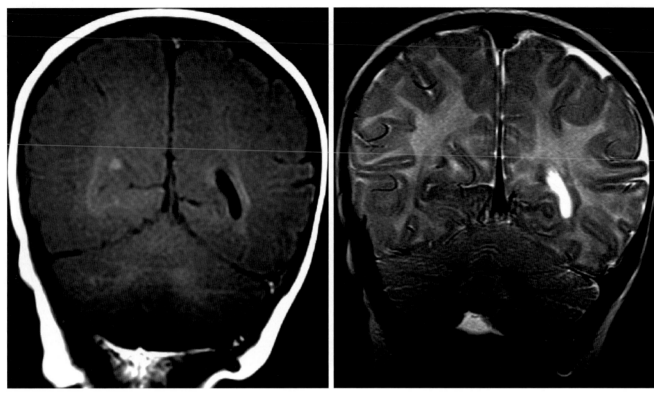

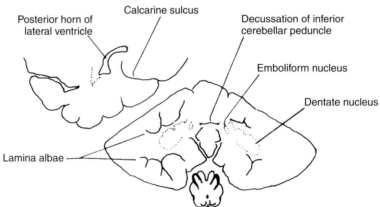

Posterior horn of
lateral ventricle

Calcarine sulcus

Decussation of inferior
cerebellar peduncle

Emboliform nucleus

Dentate nucleus

Lamina albae

POSTNATAL MR 3–4 MONTHS, CORONAL

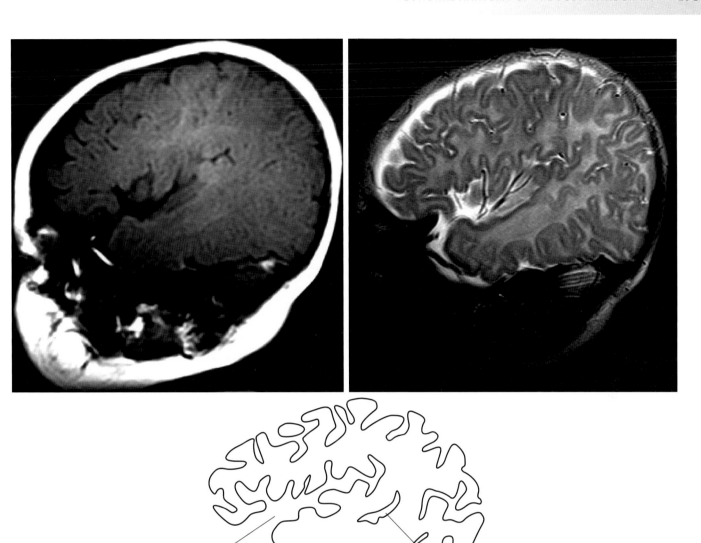

Lateral sulcus

Superior temporal sulcus

POSTNATAL MR 3–4 MONTHS, CORONAL

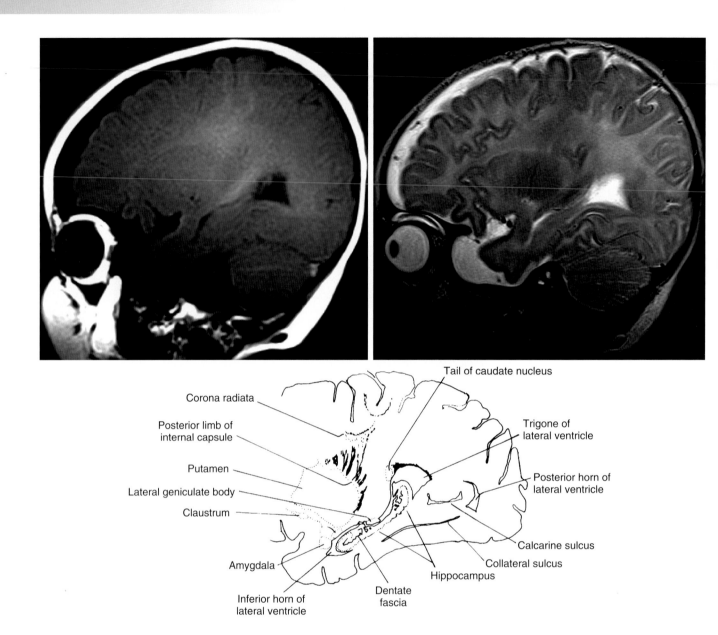

Tail of caudate nucleus

Corona radiata

Posterior limb of
internal capsule

Trigone of
lateral ventricle

Putamen

Posterior horn of
lateral ventricle

Lateral geniculate body

Claustrum

Calcarine sulcus

Amygdala

Collateral sulcus

Hippocampus

Inferior horn of
lateral ventricle

Dentate
fascia

POSTNATAL MR 3–4 MONTHS, CORONAL

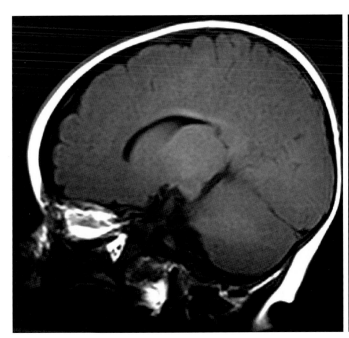
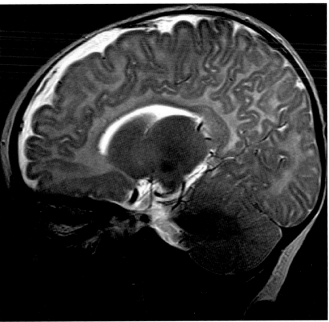

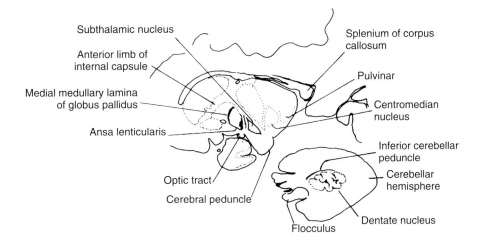

Subthalamic nucleus

Anterior limb of
internal capsule

Medial medullary lamina
of globus pallidus

Ansa lenticularis

Optic tract

Cerebral peduncle

Splenium of corpus
callosum

Pulvinar

Centromedian
nucleus

Inferior cerebellar
peduncle

Cerebellar
hemisphere

Dentate nucleus

Flocculus

POSTNATAL MR 3–4 MONTHS, SAGITTAL

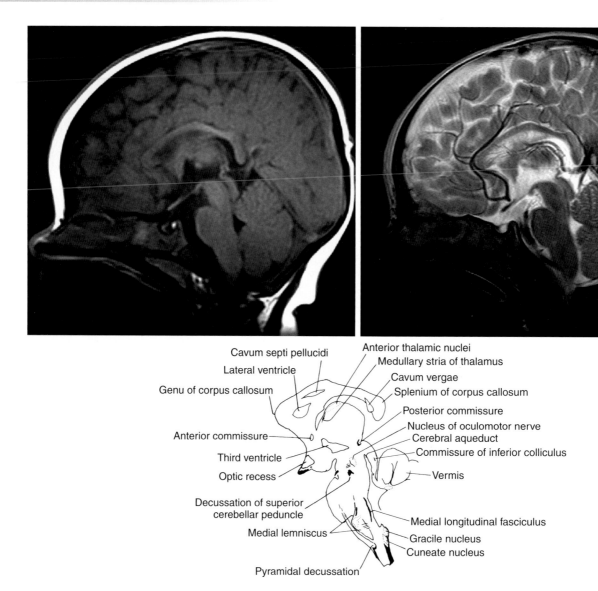

POSTNATAL MR 3–4 MONTHS, SAGITTAL

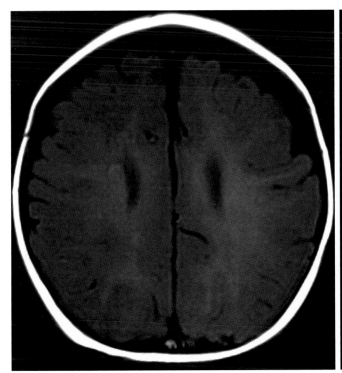
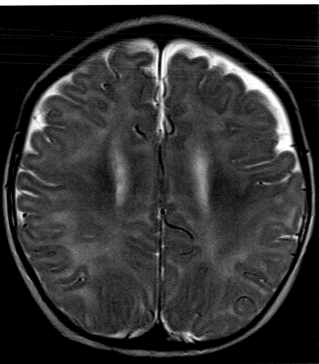

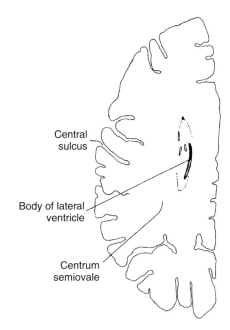

Central
sulcus

Body of lateral
ventricle

Centrum
semiovale

POSTNATAL MR 6 MONTHS, AXIAL

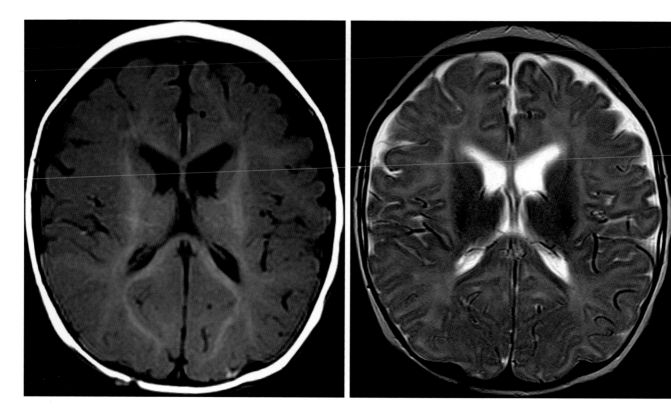

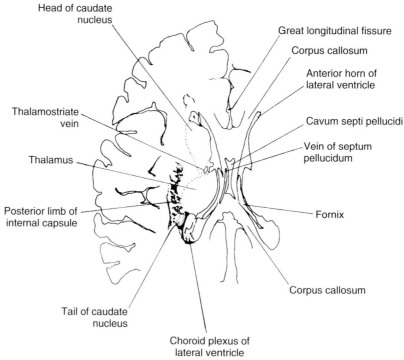

Head of caudate nucleus

Great longitudinal fissure

Corpus callosum

Anterior horn of lateral ventricle

Thalamostriate vein

Cavum septi pellucidi

Vein of septum pellucidum

Thalamus

Posterior limb of internal capsule

Fornix

Corpus callosum

Tail of caudate nucleus

Choroid plexus of lateral ventricle

POSTNATAL MR 6 MONTHS, AXIAL

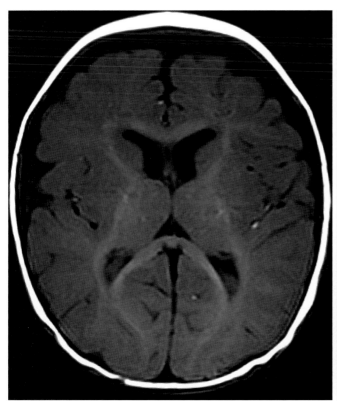
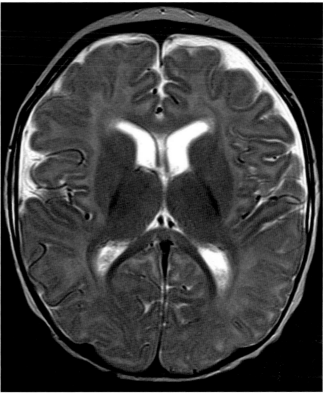

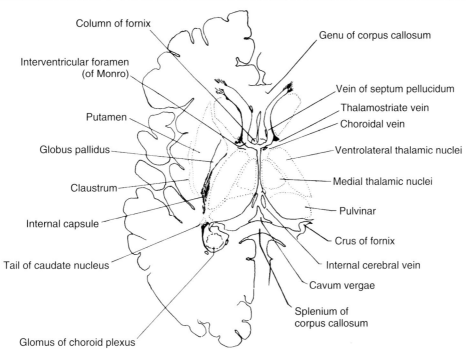

Column of fornix

Interventricular foramen (of Monro)

Putamen

Globus pallidus

Claustrum

Internal capsule

Tail of caudate nucleus

Glomus of choroid plexus

Genu of corpus callosum

Vein of septum pellucidum

Thalamostriate vein

Choroidal vein

Ventrolateral thalamic nuclei

Medial thalamic nuclei

Pulvinar

Crus of fornix

Internal cerebral vein

Cavum vergae

Splenium of corpus callosum

POSTNATAL MR 6 MONTHS, AXIAL

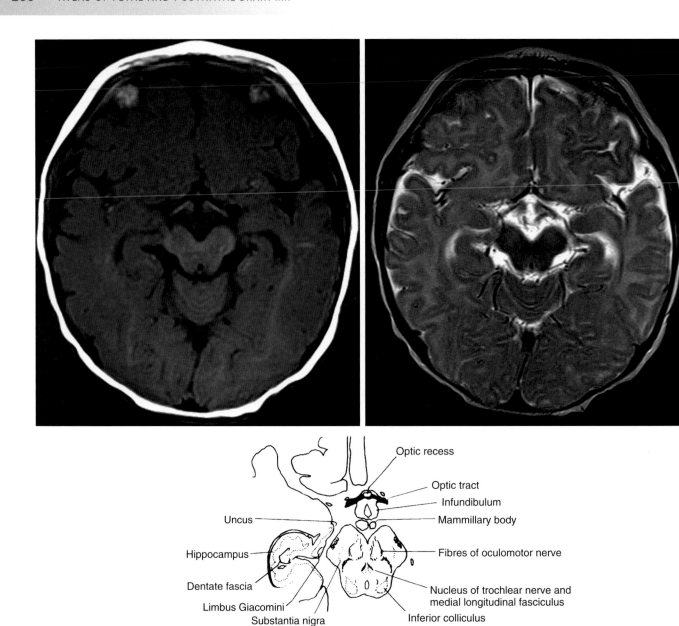

POSTNATAL MR 6 MONTHS, AXIAL

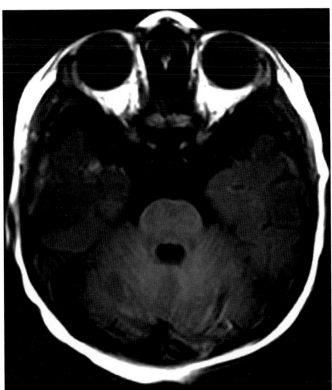
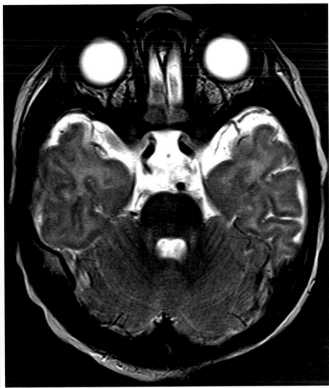

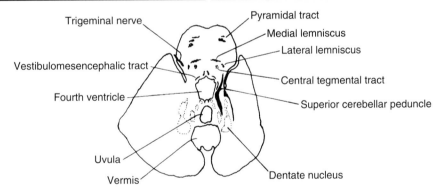

Trigeminal nerve

Vestibulomesencephalic tract

Fourth ventricle

Uvula

Vermis

Pyramidal tract

Medial lemniscus

Lateral lemniscus

Central tegmental tract

Superior cerebellar peduncle

Dentate nucleus

POSTNATAL MR 6 MONTHS, AXIAL

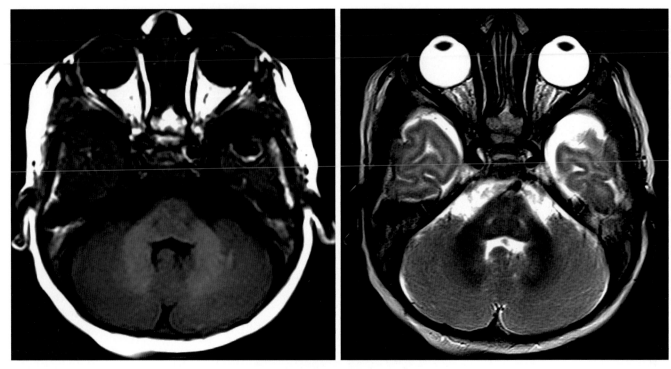

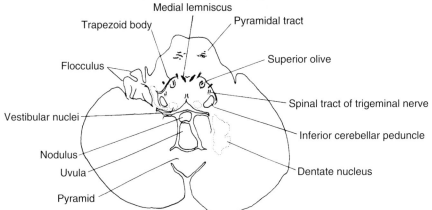

Medial lemniscus

Trapezoid body

Pyramidal tract

Flocculus

Superior olive

Vestibular nuclei

Spinal tract of trigeminal nerve

Inferior cerebellar peduncle

Nodulus

Uvula

Dentate nucleus

Pyramid

POSTNATAL MR 6 MONTHS, AXIAL

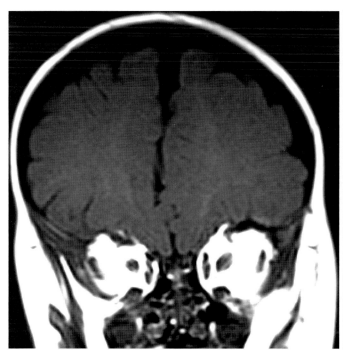
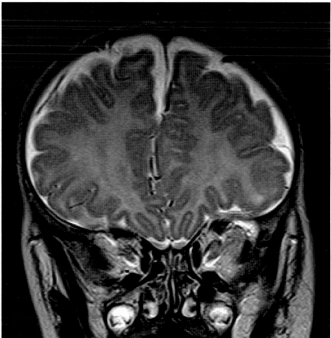

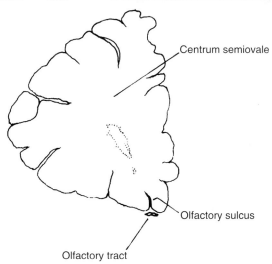

Centrum semiovale

Olfactory sulcus

Olfactory tract

POSTNATAL MR 6 MONTHS, CORONAL

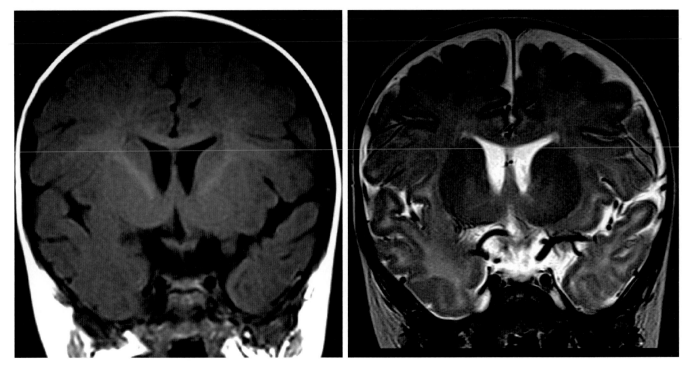

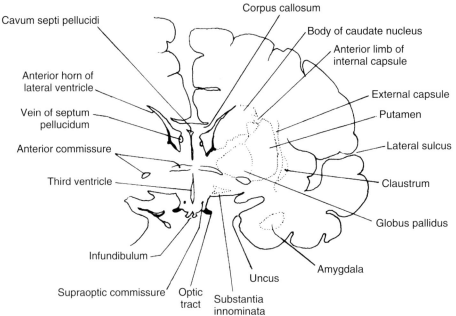

Cavum septi pellucidi

Corpus callosum

Body of caudate nucleus

Anterior limb of
internal capsule

Anterior horn of
lateral ventricle

External capsule

Vein of septum
pellucidum

Putamen

Anterior commissure

Lateral sulcus

Third ventricle

Claustrum

Globus pallidus

Infundibulum

Amygdala

Supraoptic commissure   Optic
tract

Substantia
innominata

Uncus

POSTNATAL MR 6 MONTHS, CORONAL

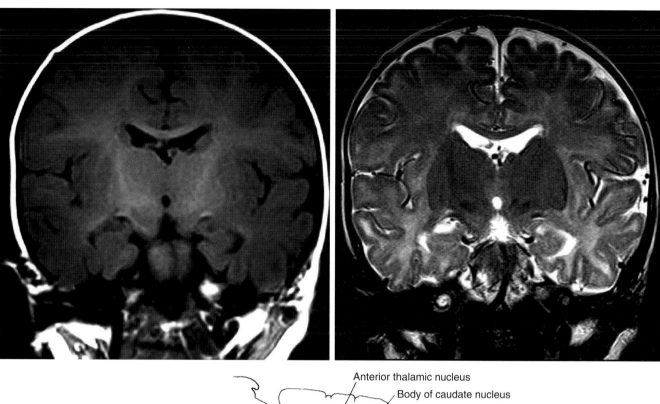

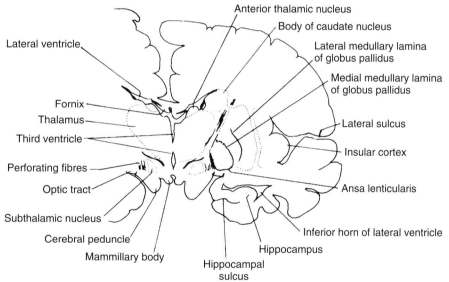

Anterior thalamic nucleus

Body of caudate nucleus

Lateral medullary lamina of globus pallidus

Medial medullary lamina of globus pallidus

Lateral ventricle

Fornix

Thalamus

Third ventricle

Perforating fibres

Optic tract

Subthalamic nucleus

Cerebral peduncle

Mammillary body

Lateral sulcus

Insular cortex

Ansa lenticularis

Inferior horn of lateral ventricle

Hippocampus

Hippocampal sulcus

POSTNATAL MR 6 MONTHS, CORONAL

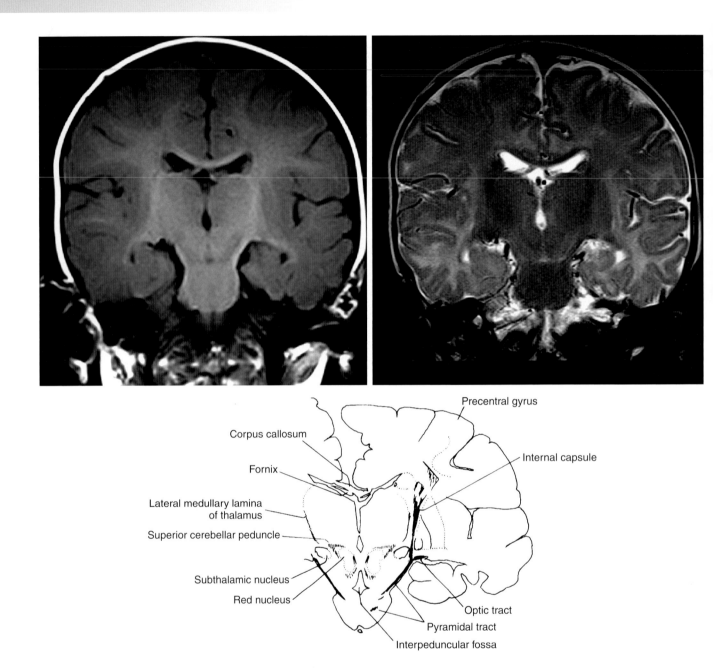

POSTNATAL MR 6 MONTHS, CORONAL

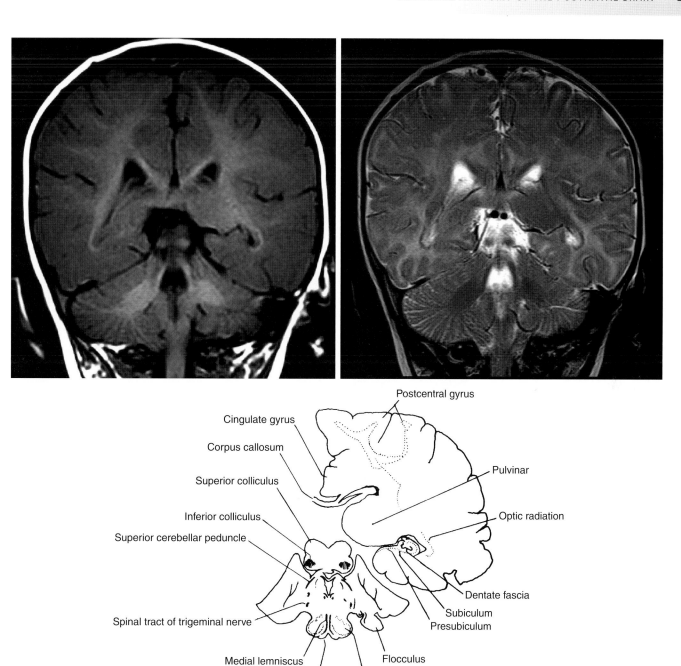

Postcentral gyrus

Cingulate gyrus

Corpus callosum

Superior colliculus

Pulvinar

Inferior colliculus

Optic radiation

Superior cerebellar peduncle

Dentate fascia

Subiculum

Presubiculum

Spinal tract of trigeminal nerve

Medial lemniscus

Flocculus

Pyramid

Inferior olive

POSTNATAL MR 6 MONTHS, CORONAL

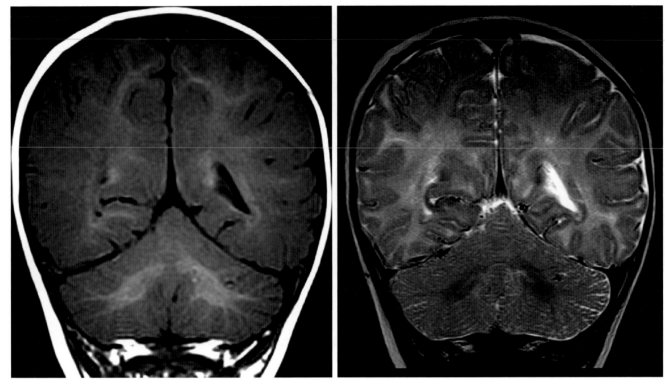

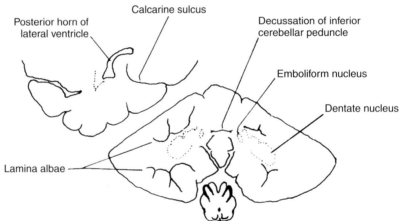

Posterior horn of
lateral ventricle

Calcarine sulcus

Decussation of inferior
cerebellar peduncle

Emboliform nucleus

Dentate nucleus

Lamina albae

POSTNATAL MR 6 MONTHS, CORONAL

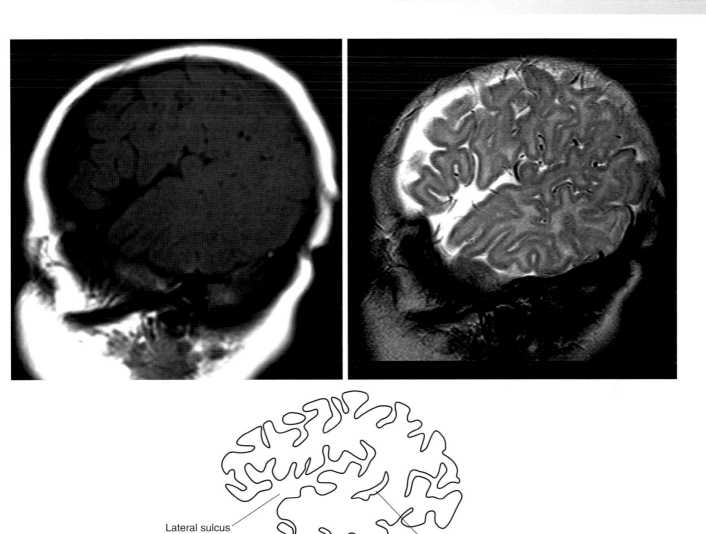

Lateral sulcus

Superior temporal sulcus

POSTNATAL MR 6 MONTHS, SAGITTAL

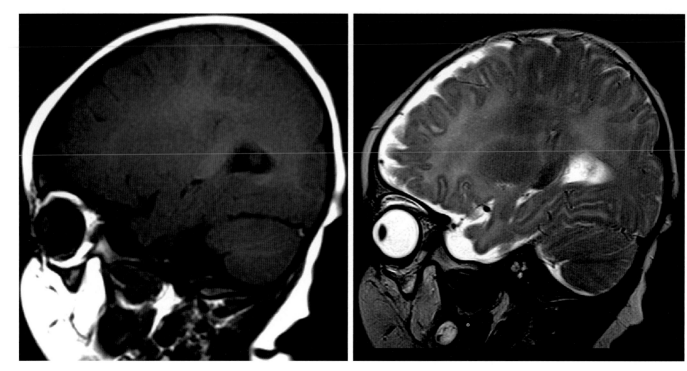

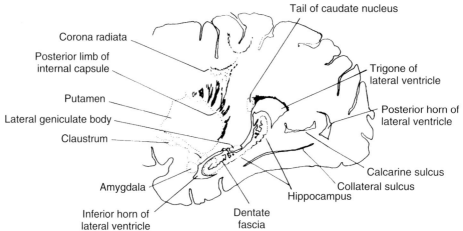

Corona radiata

Posterior limb of
internal capsule

Putamen

Lateral geniculate body

Claustrum

Amygdala

Inferior horn of
lateral ventricle

Dentate
fascia

Hippocampus

Collateral sulcus

Calcarine sulcus

Posterior horn of
lateral ventricle

Trigone of
lateral ventricle

Tail of caudate nucleus

POSTNATAL MR 6 MONTHS, SAGITTAL

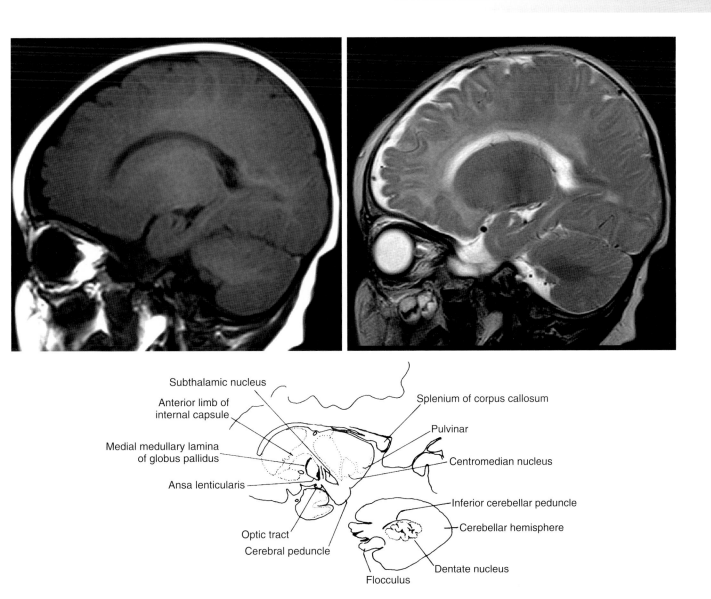

Subthalamic nucleus

Anterior limb of
internal capsule

Medial medullary lamina
of globus pallidus

Ansa lenticularis

Optic tract

Cerebral peduncle

Splenium of corpus callosum

Pulvinar

Centromedian nucleus

Inferior cerebellar peduncle

Cerebellar hemisphere

Dentate nucleus

Flocculus

POSTNATAL MR 6 MONTHS, SAGITTAL

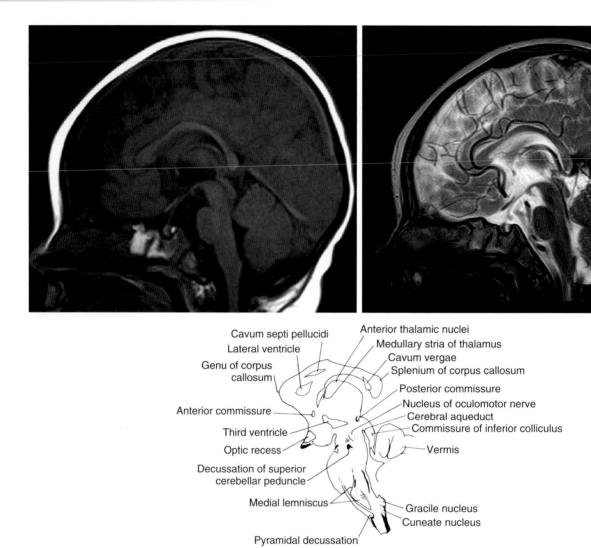

Cavum septi pellucidi
Lateral ventricle
Genu of corpus callosum
Anterior commissure
Third ventricle
Optic recess
Decussation of superior cerebellar peduncle
Medial lemniscus
Pyramidal decussation

Anterior thalamic nuclei
Medullary stria of thalamus
Cavum vergae
Splenium of corpus callosum
Posterior commissure
Nucleus of oculomotor nerve
Cerebral aqueduct
Commissure of inferior colliculus
Vermis
Gracile nucleus
Cuneate nucleus

POSTNATAL MR 6 MONTHS, SAGITTAL

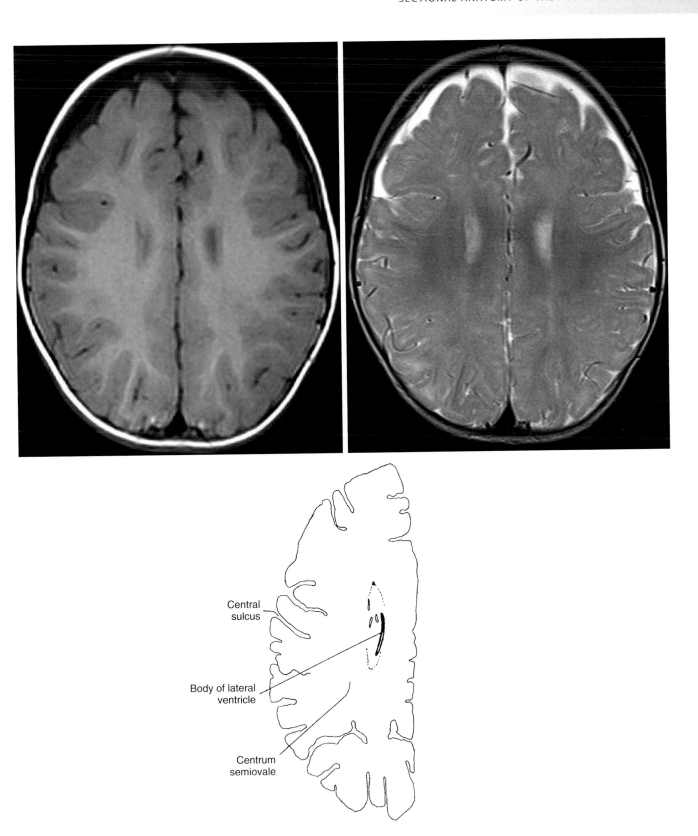

Central
sulcus

Body of lateral
ventricle

Centrum
semiovale

POSTNATAL MR 9 MONTHS, AXIAL

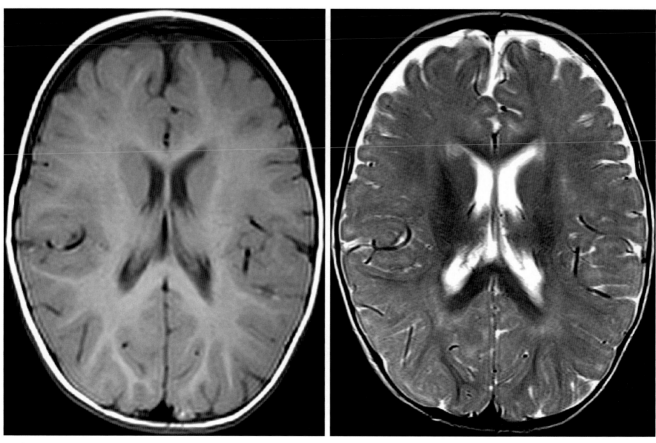

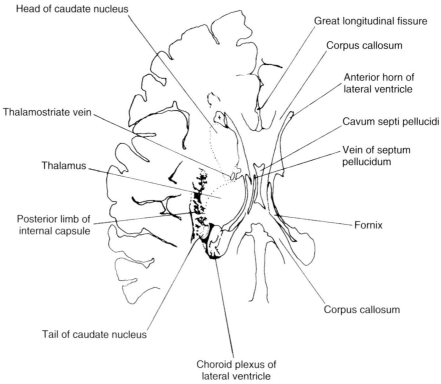

Head of caudate nucleus

Great longitudinal fissure

Corpus callosum

Anterior horn of
lateral ventricle

Thalamostriate vein

Cavum septi pellucidi

Vein of septum
pellucidum

Thalamus

Posterior limb of
internal capsule

Fornix

Corpus callosum

Tail of caudate nucleus

Choroid plexus of
lateral ventricle

POSTNATAL MR 9 MONTHS, AXIAL

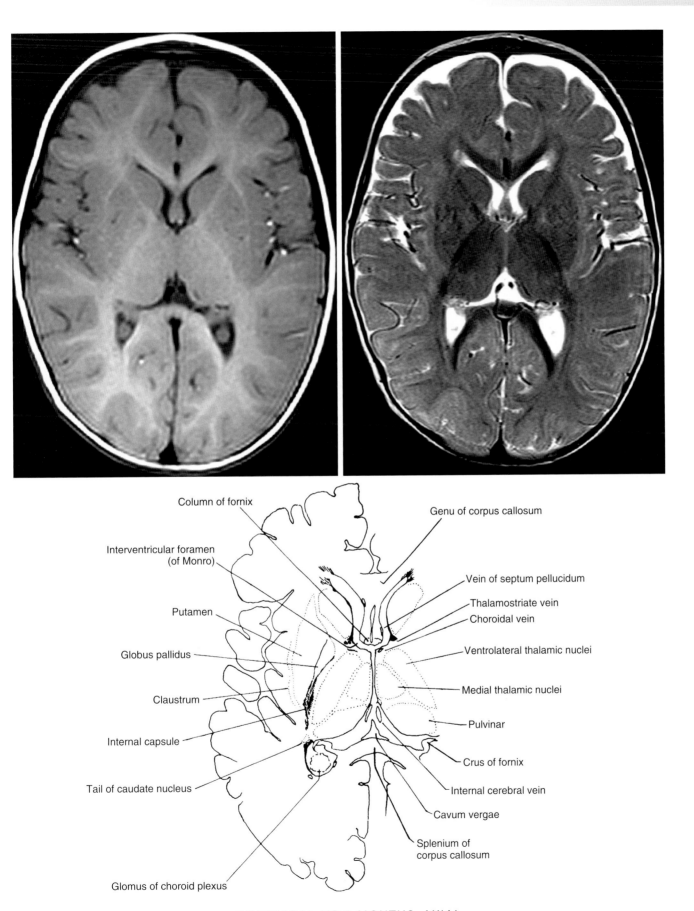

Column of fornix

Interventricular foramen
(of Monro)

Putamen

Globus pallidus

Claustrum

Internal capsule

Tail of caudate nucleus

Glomus of choroid plexus

Genu of corpus callosum

Vein of septum pellucidum

Thalamostriate vein

Choroidal vein

Ventrolateral thalamic nuclei

Medial thalamic nuclei

Pulvinar

Crus of fornix

Internal cerebral vein

Cavum vergae

Splenium of
corpus callosum

POSTNATAL MR 9 MONTHS, AXIAL

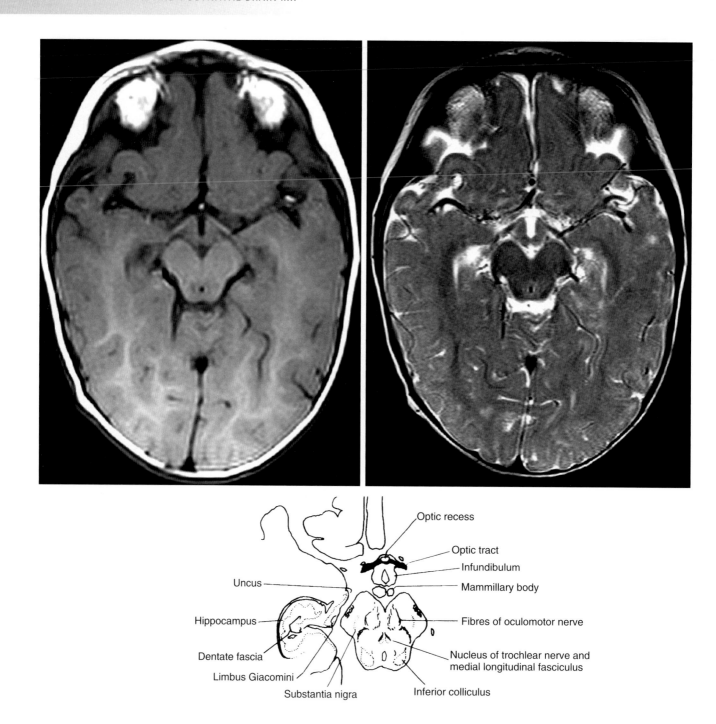

POSTNATAL MR 9 MONTHS, AXIAL

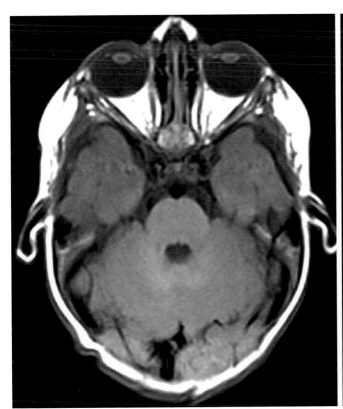
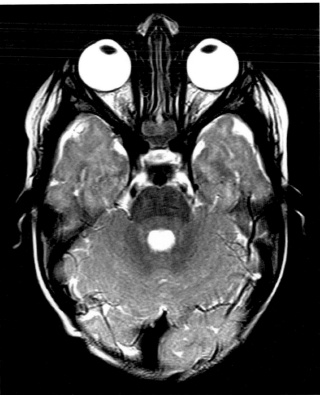

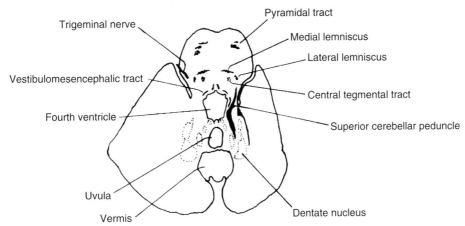

Trigeminal nerve

Pyramidal tract

Medial lemniscus

Lateral lemniscus

Vestibulomesencephalic tract

Central tegmental tract

Fourth ventricle

Superior cerebellar peduncle

Uvula

Vermis

Dentate nucleus

POSTNATAL MR 9 MONTHS, AXIAL

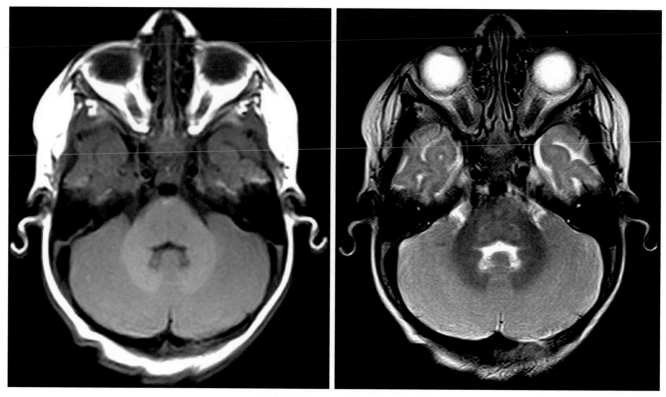

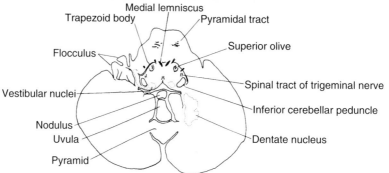

POSTNATAL MR 9 MONTHS, AXIAL

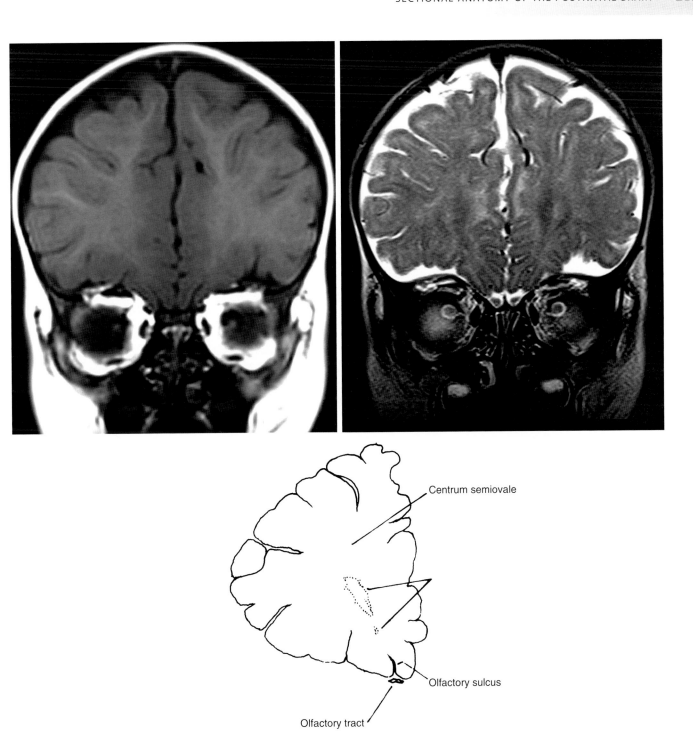

Centrum semiovale

Olfactory sulcus

Olfactory tract

POSTNATAL MR 9 MONTHS, CORONAL

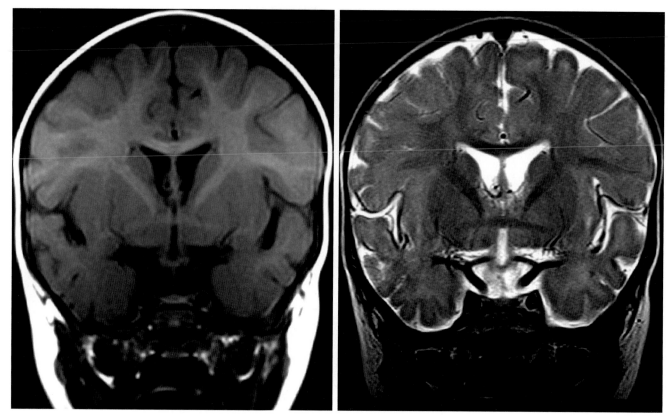

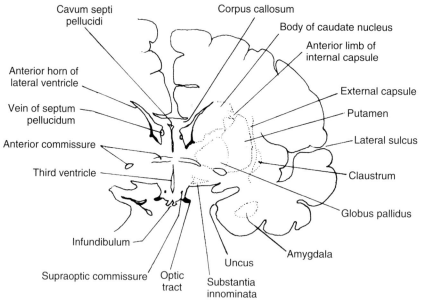

Cavum septi
pellucidi

Corpus callosum

Body of caudate nucleus

Anterior limb of
internal capsule

Anterior horn of
lateral ventricle

External capsule

Putamen

Vein of septum
pellucidum

Lateral sulcus

Anterior commissure

Claustrum

Third ventricle

Globus pallidus

Infundibulum

Amygdala

Supraoptic commissure   Optic
tract

Uncus

Substantia
innominata

POSTNATAL MR 9 MONTHS, CORONAL

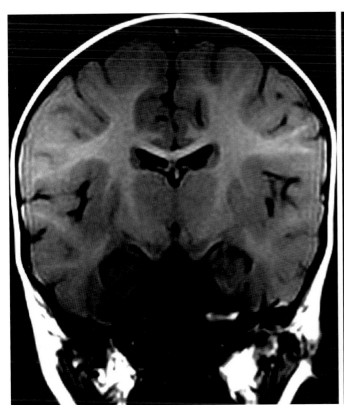
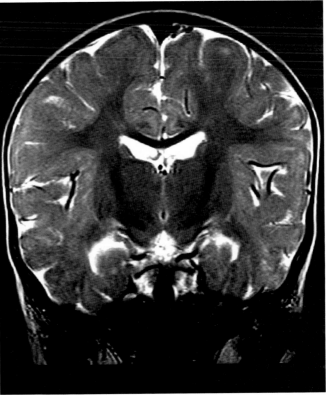

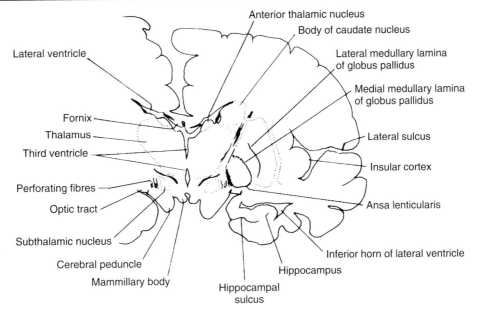

Anterior thalamic nucleus

Body of caudate nucleus

Lateral ventricle

Lateral medullary lamina
of globus pallidus

Medial medullary lamina
of globus pallidus

Fornix

Thalamus

Lateral sulcus

Third ventricle

Insular cortex

Perforating fibres

Optic tract

Ansa lenticularis

Subthalamic nucleus

Cerebral peduncle

Inferior horn of lateral ventricle

Mammillary body

Hippocampus

Hippocampal
sulcus

POSTNATAL MR 9 MONTHS, CORONAL

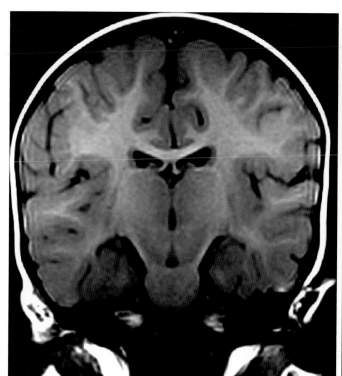
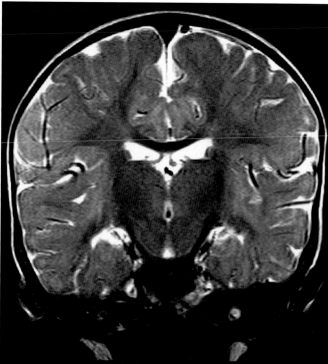

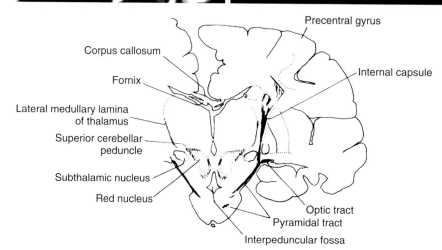

Precentral gyrus

Corpus callosum

Fornix

Internal capsule

Lateral medullary lamina
of thalamus

Superior cerebellar
peduncle

Subthalamic nucleus

Red nucleus

Optic tract

Pyramidal tract

Interpeduncular fossa

POSTNATAL MR 9 MONTHS, CORONAL

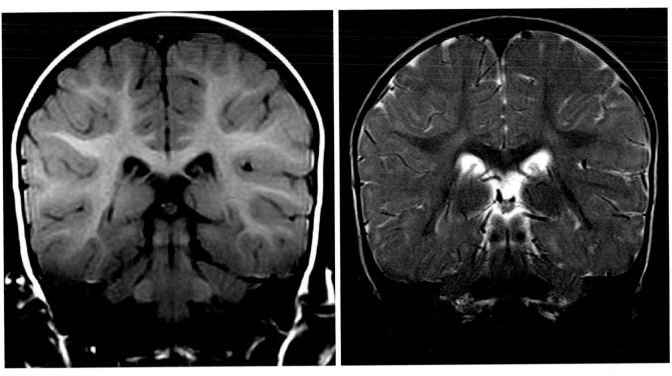

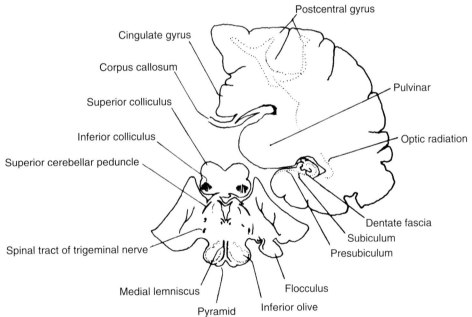

Postcentral gyrus

Cingulate gyrus

Corpus callosum

Superior colliculus

Inferior colliculus

Superior cerebellar peduncle

Pulvinar

Optic radiation

Spinal tract of trigeminal nerve

Dentate fascia

Subiculum

Presubiculum

Medial lemniscus

Flocculus

Pyramid

Inferior olive

POSTNATAL MR 9 MONTHS, CORONAL

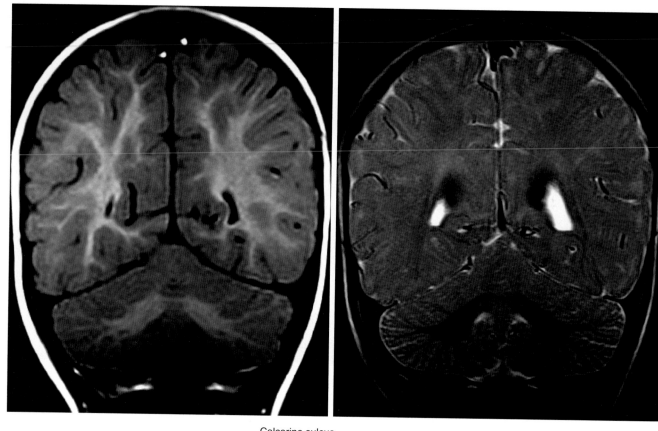

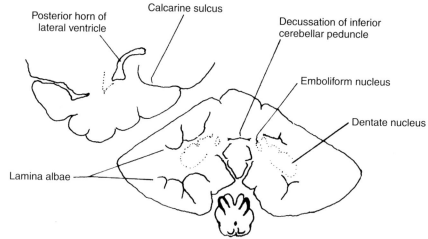

Posterior horn of lateral ventricle

Calcarine sulcus

Decussation of inferior cerebellar peduncle

Emboliform nucleus

Dentate nucleus

Lamina albae

POSTNATAL MR 9 MONTHS, CORONAL

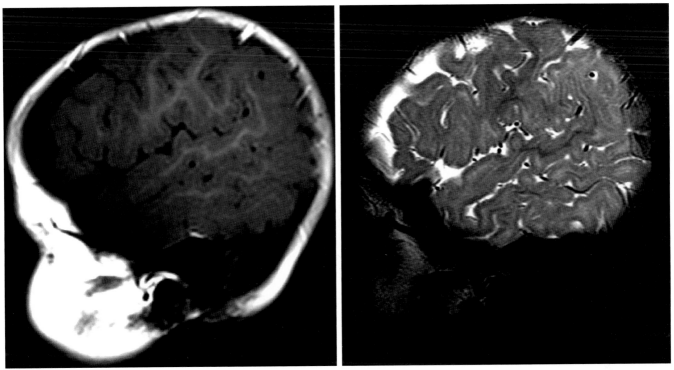

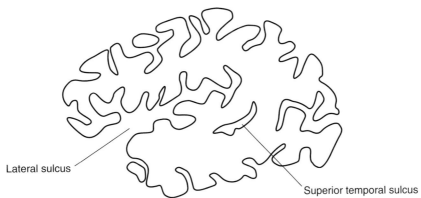

Lateral sulcus

Superior temporal sulcus

POSTNATAL MR 9 MONTHS, SAGITTAL

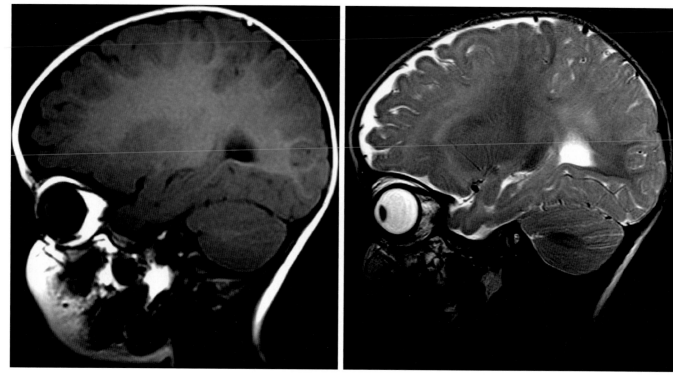

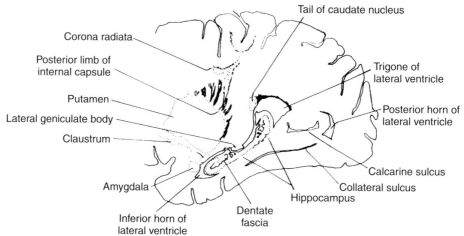

Tail of caudate nucleus

Corona radiata

Posterior limb of
internal capsule

Trigone of
lateral ventricle

Putamen

Posterior horn of
lateral ventricle

Lateral geniculate body

Claustrum

Amygdala

Calcarine sulcus

Collateral sulcus

Hippocampus

Inferior horn of
lateral ventricle

Dentate
fascia

POSTNATAL MR 9 MONTHS, SAGITTAL

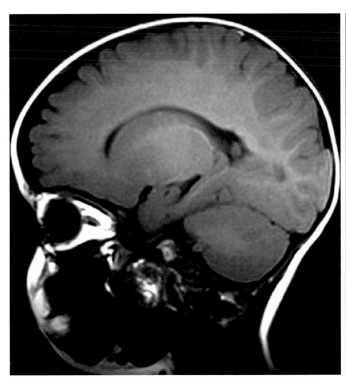
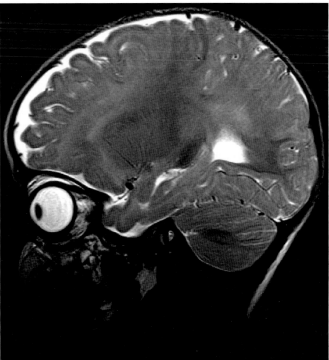

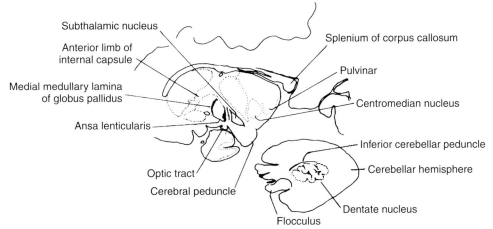

Subthalamic nucleus

Anterior limb of
internal capsule

Medial medullary lamina
of globus pallidus

Ansa lenticularis

Optic tract

Cerebral peduncle

Splenium of corpus callosum

Pulvinar

Centromedian nucleus

Inferior cerebellar peduncle

Cerebellar hemisphere

Dentate nucleus

Flocculus

POSTNATAL MR 9 MONTHS, SAGITTAL

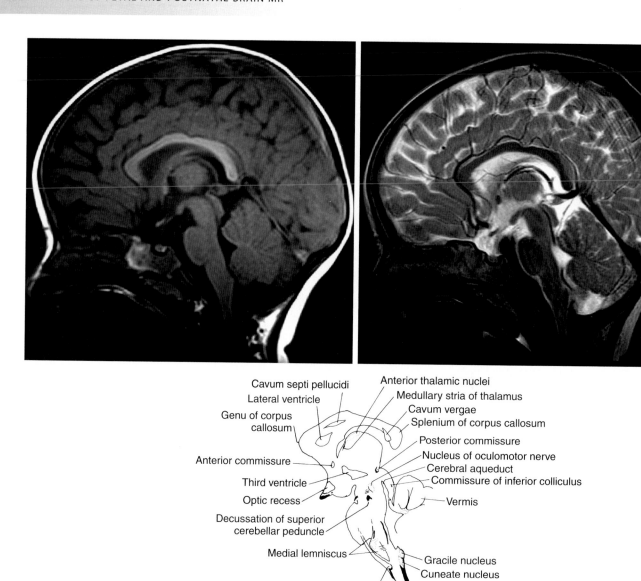

Cavum septi pellucidi
Lateral ventricle
Genu of corpus callosum
Anterior commissure
Third ventricle
Optic recess
Decussation of superior cerebellar peduncle
Medial lemniscus
Pyramidal decussation

Anterior thalamic nuclei
Medullary stria of thalamus
Cavum vergae
Splenium of corpus callosum
Posterior commissure
Nucleus of oculomotor nerve
Cerebral aqueduct
Commissure of inferior colliculus
Vermis
Gracile nucleus
Cuneate nucleus

POSTNATAL MR 9 MONTHS, SAGITTAL

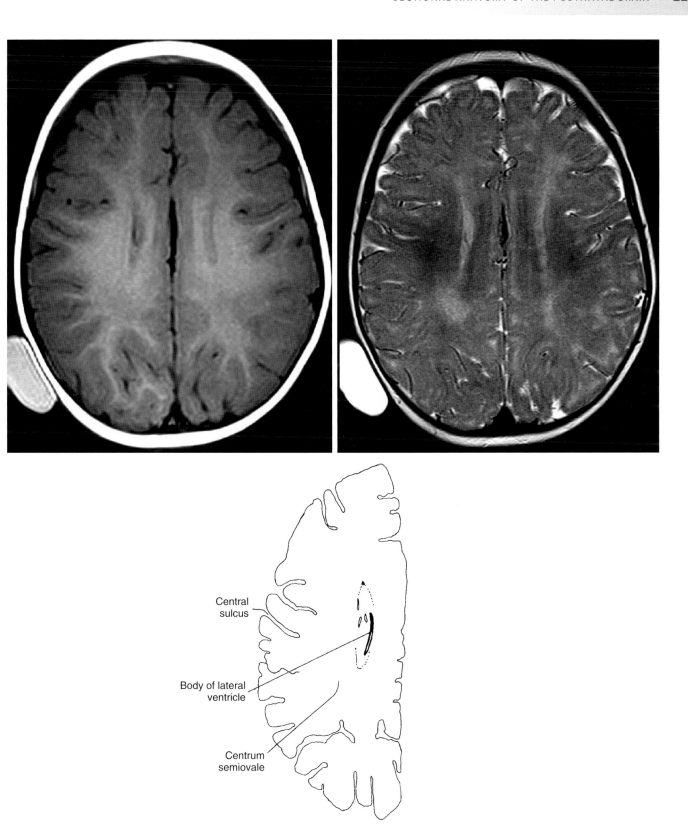

Central
sulcus

Body of lateral
ventricle

Centrum
semiovale

POSTNATAL MR 12 MONTHS, AXIAL

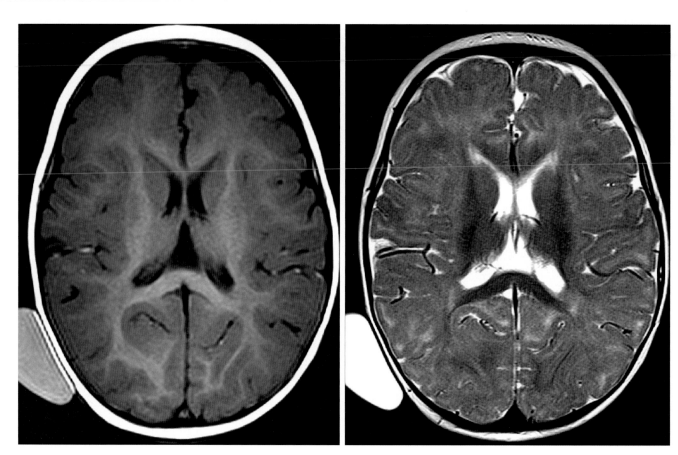

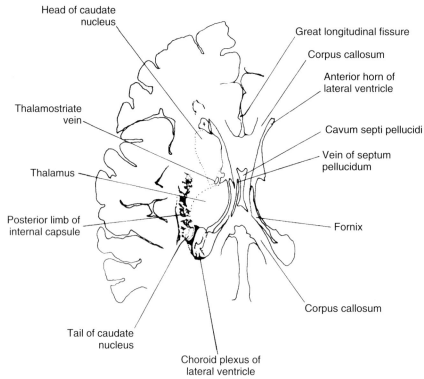

Head of caudate
nucleus

Great longitudinal fissure

Corpus callosum

Anterior horn of
lateral ventricle

Thalamostriate
vein

Cavum septi pellucidi

Vein of septum
pellucidum

Thalamus

Posterior limb of
internal capsule

Fornix

Corpus callosum

Tail of caudate
nucleus

Choroid plexus of
lateral ventricle

POSTNATAL MR 12 MONTHS, AXIAL

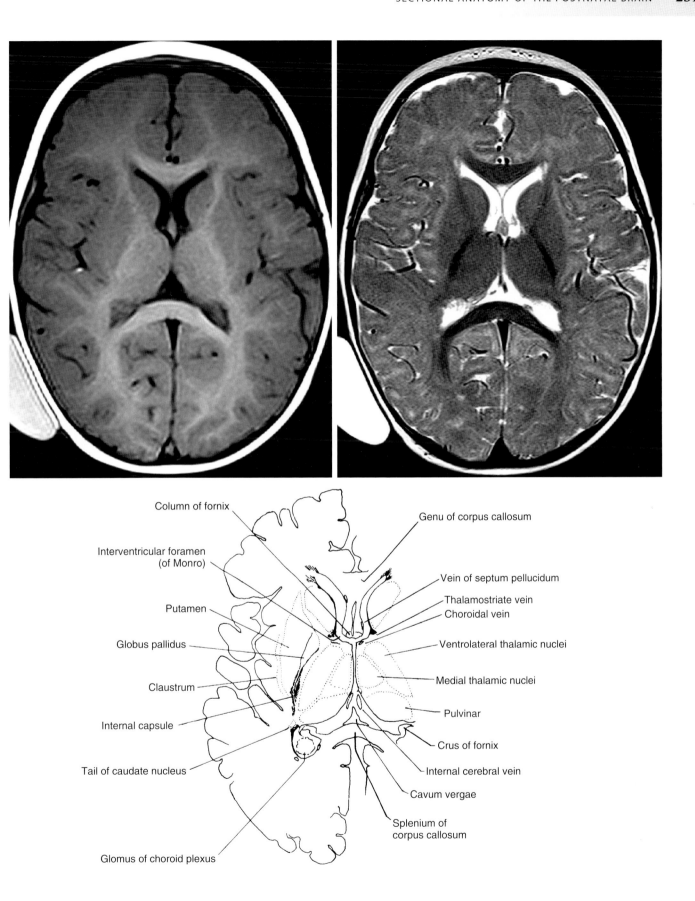

Column of fornix

Interventricular foramen
(of Monro)

Putamen

Globus pallidus

Claustrum

Internal capsule

Tail of caudate nucleus

Glomus of choroid plexus

Genu of corpus callosum

Vein of septum pellucidum

Thalamostriate vein
Choroidal vein

Ventrolateral thalamic nuclei

Medial thalamic nuclei

Pulvinar

Crus of fornix

Internal cerebral vein

Cavum vergae

Splenium of
corpus callosum

POSTNATAL MR 12 MONTHS, AXIAL

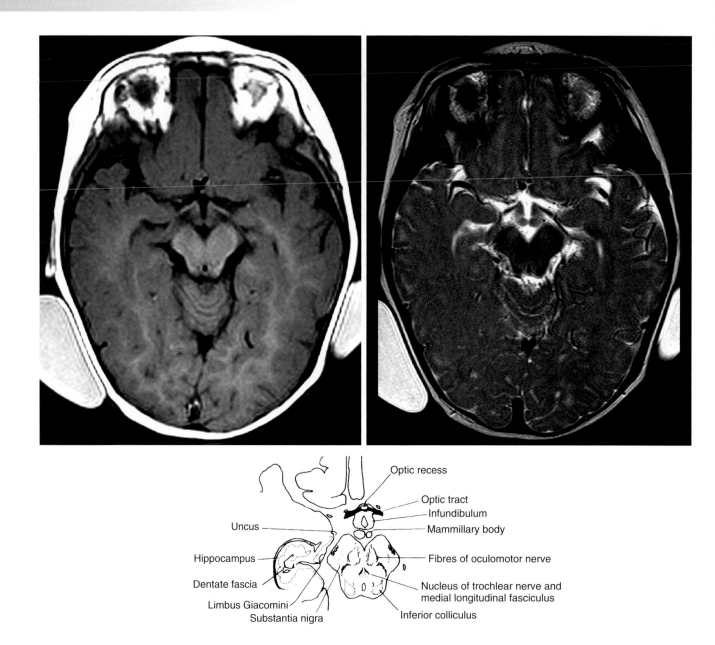

POSTNATAL MR 12 MONTHS, AXIAL

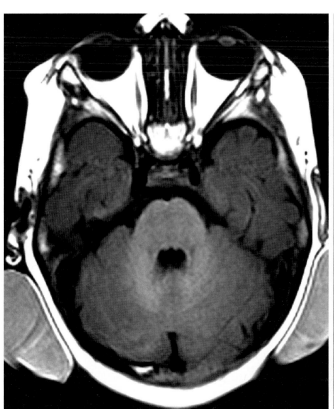
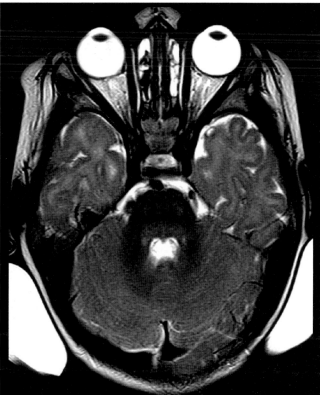

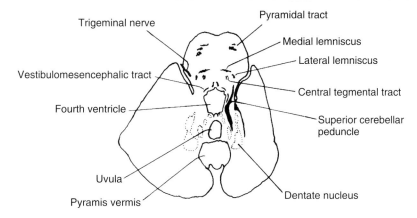

Trigeminal nerve

Pyramidal tract

Medial lemniscus

Lateral lemniscus

Vestibulomesencephalic tract

Central tegmental tract

Fourth ventricle

Superior cerebellar peduncle

Uvula

Dentate nucleus

Pyramis vermis

POSTNATAL MR 12 MONTHS, AXIAL

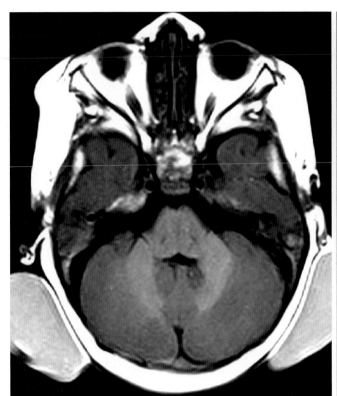
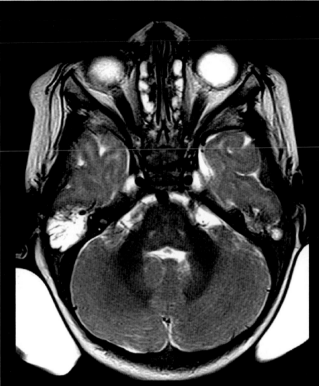

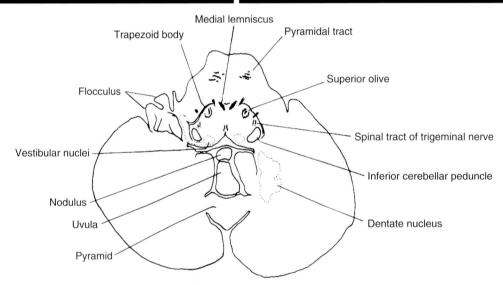

Trapezoid body · Medial lemniscus · Pyramidal tract

Flocculus

Superior olive

Spinal tract of trigeminal nerve

Vestibular nuclei

Inferior cerebellar peduncle

Nodulus

Uvula

Dentate nucleus

Pyramid

POSTNATAL MR 12 MONTHS, AXIAL

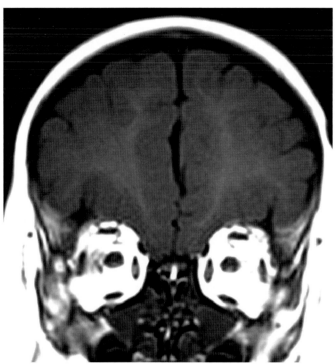
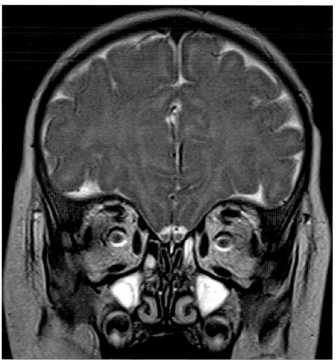

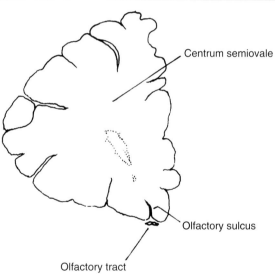

Centrum semiovale

Olfactory sulcus

Olfactory tract

POSTNATAL MR 12 MONTHS, CORONAL

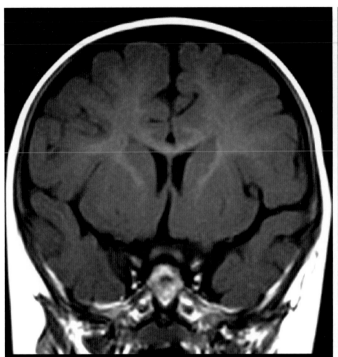
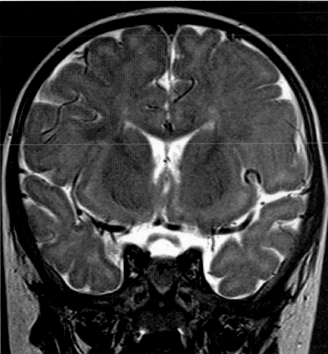
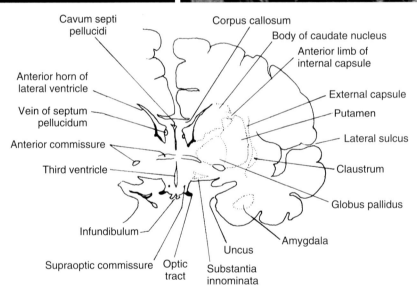

Cavum septi pellucidi

Corpus callosum

Body of caudate nucleus

Anterior limb of internal capsule

Anterior horn of lateral ventricle

Vein of septum pellucidum

External capsule

Putamen

Anterior commissure

Lateral sulcus

Third ventricle

Claustrum

Globus pallidus

Infundibulum

Amygdala

Supraoptic commissure

Optic tract

Substantia innominata

Uncus

POSTNATAL MR 12 MONTHS, CORONAL

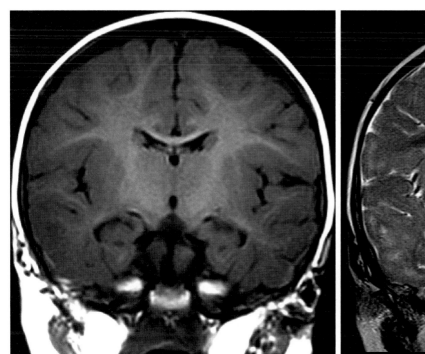
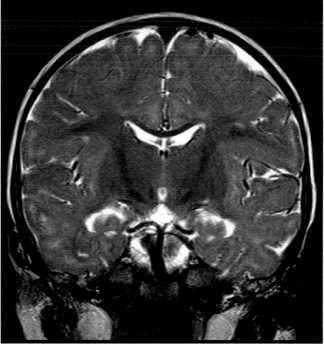

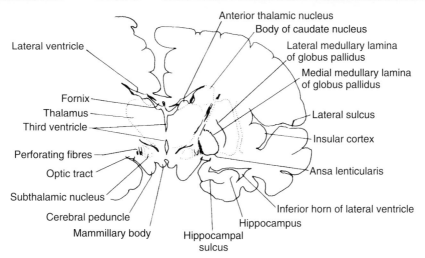

Anterior thalamic nucleus
Body of caudate nucleus
Lateral ventricle
Lateral medullary lamina of globus pallidus
Medial medullary lamina of globus pallidus
Fornix
Thalamus
Third ventricle
Lateral sulcus
Insular cortex
Perforating fibres
Optic tract
Ansa lenticularis
Subthalamic nucleus
Cerebral peduncle
Inferior horn of lateral ventricle
Mammillary body
Hippocampus
Hippocampal sulcus

POSTNATAL MR 12 MONTHS, CORONAL

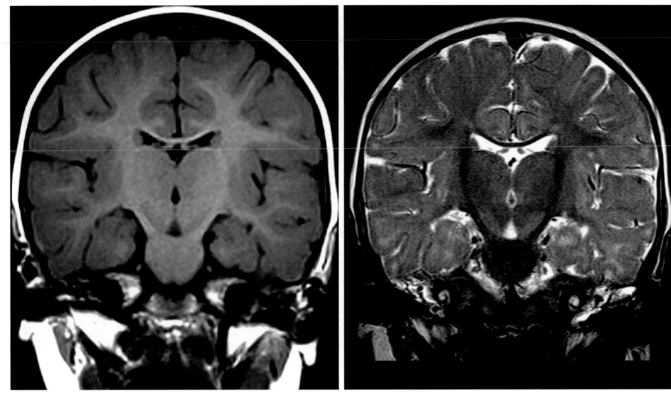

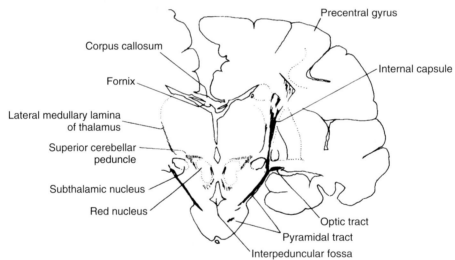

Precentral gyrus

Corpus callosum

Internal capsule

Fornix

Lateral medullary lamina
of thalamus

Superior cerebellar
peduncle

Subthalamic nucleus

Red nucleus

Optic tract

Pyramidal tract

Interpeduncular fossa

POSTNATAL MR 12 MONTHS, CORONAL

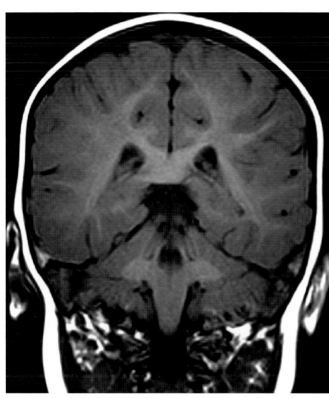
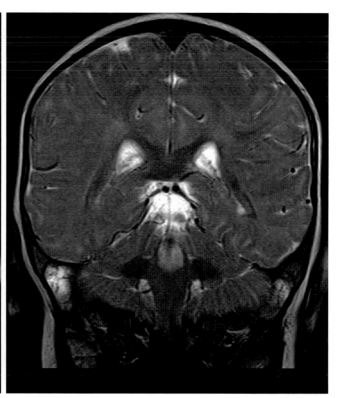

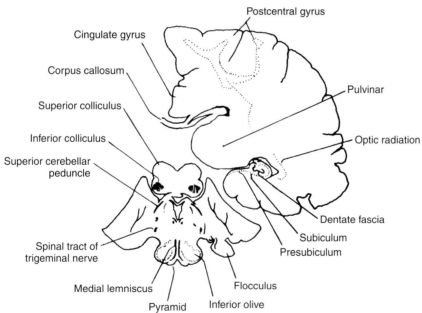

Postcentral gyrus

Cingulate gyrus

Corpus callosum

Superior colliculus

Inferior colliculus

Superior cerebellar
peduncle

Pulvinar

Optic radiation

Dentate fascia

Subiculum

Presubiculum

Spinal tract of
trigeminal nerve

Medial lemniscus

Pyramid

Flocculus

Inferior olive

POSTNATAL MR 12 MONTHS, CORONAL

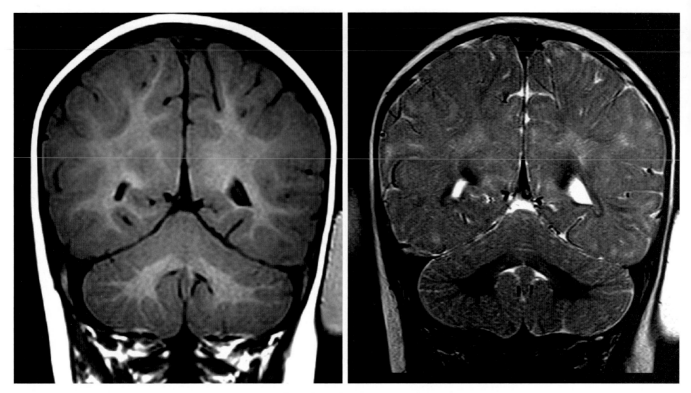

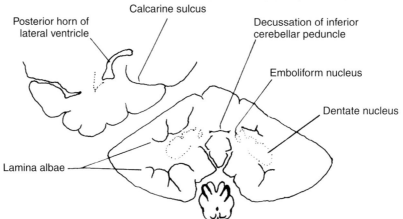

Posterior horn of
lateral ventricle

Calcarine sulcus

Decussation of inferior
cerebellar peduncle

Emboliform nucleus

Dentate nucleus

Lamina albae

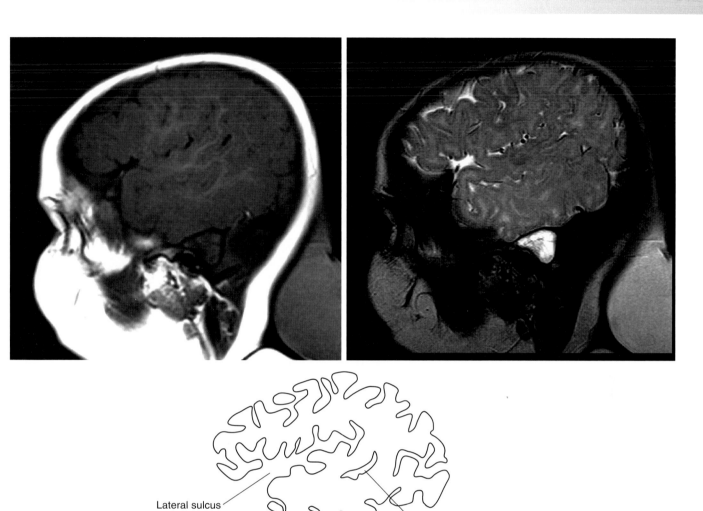

Lateral sulcus

Superior temporal sulcus

POSTNATAL MR 12 MONTHS, SAGITTAL

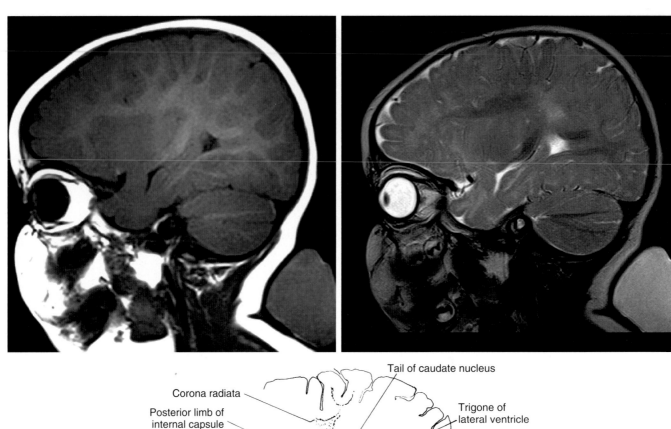

Corona radiata

Posterior limb of
internal capsule

Putamen

Lateral geniculate body

Claustrum

Amygdala

Inferior horn of
lateral ventricle

Dentate
fascia

Hippocampus

Collateral sulcus

Calcarine sulcus

Posterior horn of
lateral ventricle

Trigone of
lateral ventricle

Tail of caudate nucleus

POSTNATAL MR 12 MONTHS, SAGITTAL

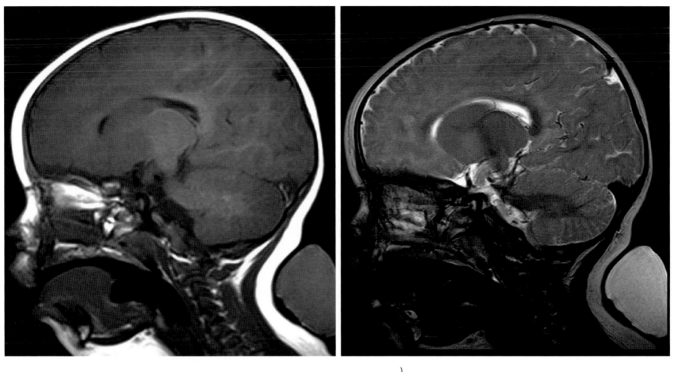

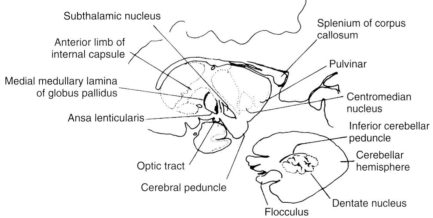

Subthalamic nucleus

Anterior limb of
internal capsule

Medial medullary lamina
of globus pallidus

Ansa lenticularis

Optic tract

Cerebral peduncle

Splenium of corpus
callosum

Pulvinar

Centromedian
nucleus

Inferior cerebellar
peduncle

Cerebellar
hemisphere

Dentate nucleus

Flocculus

POSTNATAL MR 12 MONTHS, SAGITTAL

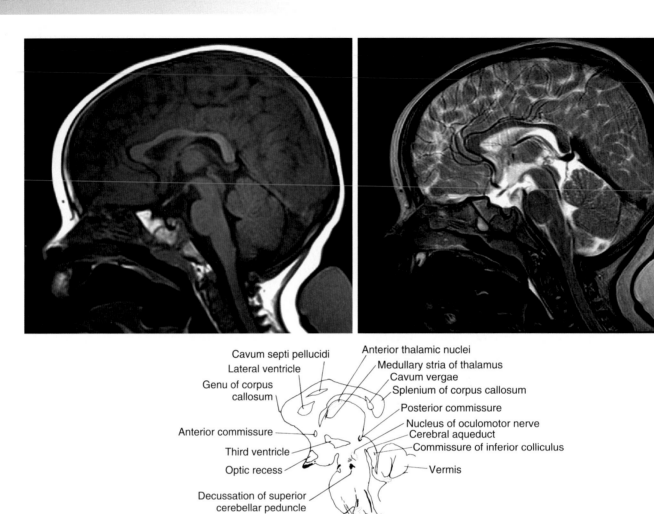

Cavum septi pellucidi
Lateral ventricle
Genu of corpus callosum
Anterior commissure
Third ventricle
Optic recess
Decussation of superior cerebellar peduncle
Medial lemniscus
Pyramidal decussation

Anterior thalamic nuclei
Medullary stria of thalamus
Cavum vergae
Splenium of corpus callosum
Posterior commissure
Nucleus of oculomotor nerve
Cerebral aqueduct
Commissure of inferior colliculus
Vermis
Gracile nucleus
Cuneate nucleus

POSTNATAL MR 12 MONTHS, SAGITTAL

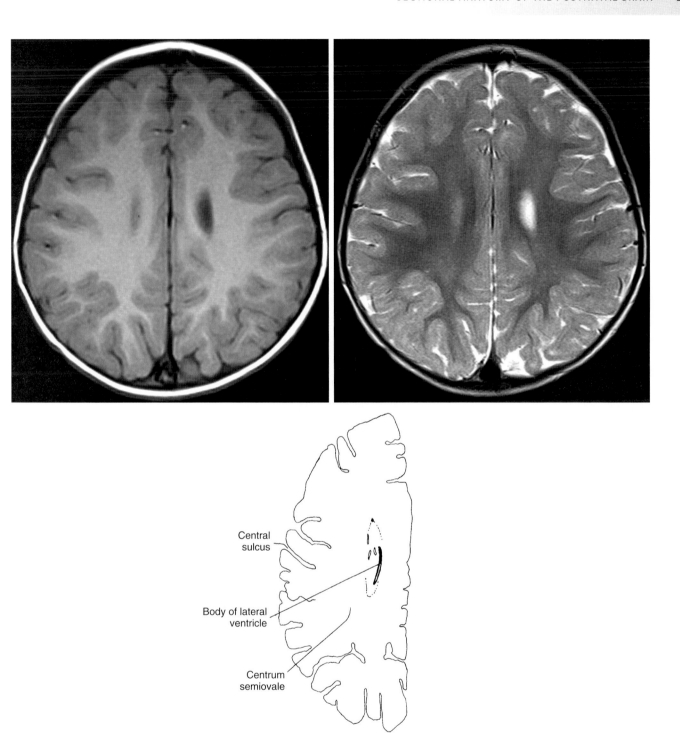

Central
sulcus

Body of lateral
ventricle

Centrum
semiovale

POSTNATAL MR 18 MONTHS, AXIAL

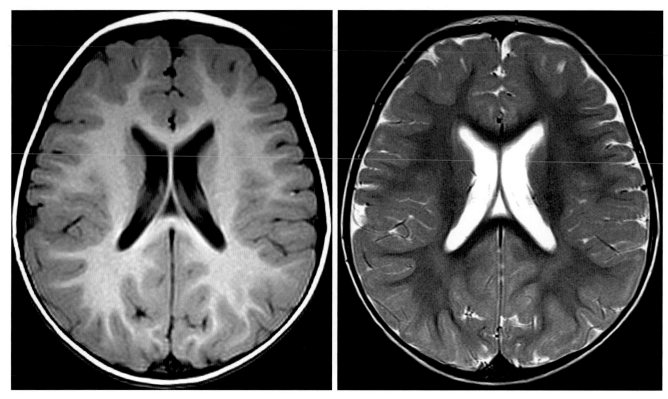

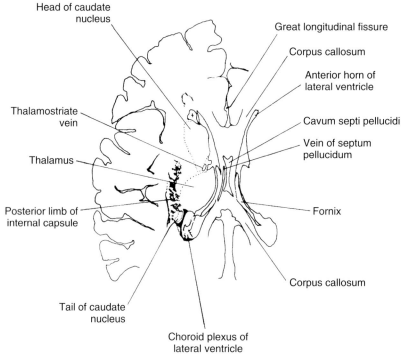

Head of caudate
nucleus

Great longitudinal fissure

Corpus callosum

Anterior horn of
lateral ventricle

Thalamostriate
vein

Cavum septi pellucidi

Vein of septum
pellucidum

Thalamus

Posterior limb of
internal capsule

Fornix

Corpus callosum

Tail of caudate
nucleus

Choroid plexus of
lateral ventricle

POSTNATAL MR 18 MONTHS, AXIAL

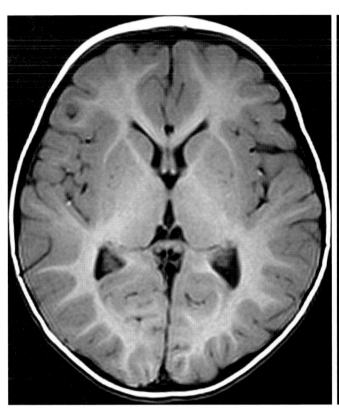
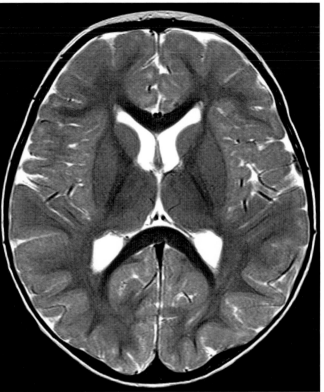

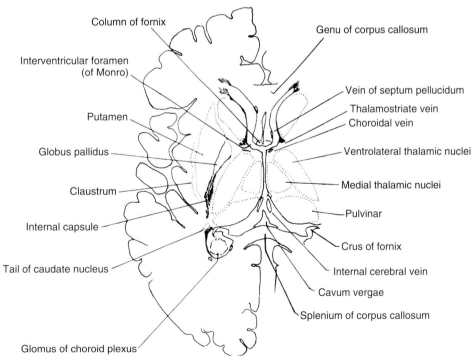

Column of fornix

Interventricular foramen
(of Monro)

Putamen

Globus pallidus

Claustrum

Internal capsule

Tail of caudate nucleus

Glomus of choroid plexus

Genu of corpus callosum

Vein of septum pellucidum
Thalamostriate vein
Choroidal vein

Ventrolateral thalamic nuclei

Medial thalamic nuclei

Pulvinar

Crus of fornix

Internal cerebral vein

Cavum vergae

Splenium of corpus callosum

POSTNATAL MR 18 MONTHS, AXIAL

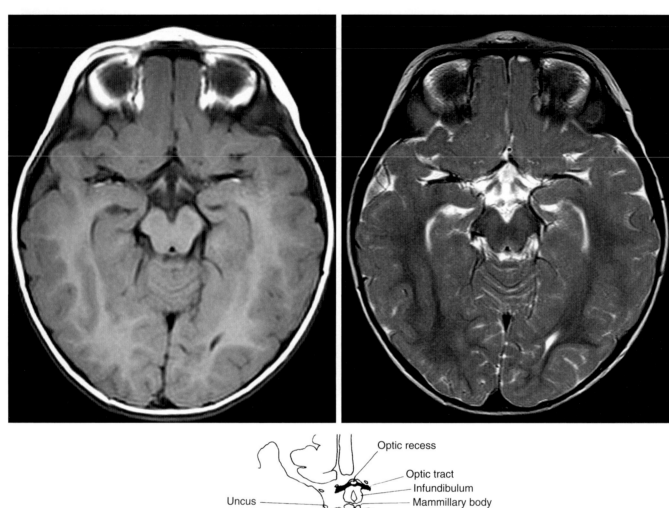

Optic recess

Optic tract

Infundibulum

Uncus

Mammillary body

Hippocampus

Fibres of oculomotor nerve

Dentate fascia

Nucleus of trochlear nerve and
medial longitudinal fasciculus

Limbus Giacomini

Substantia nigra

Inferior colliculus

POSTNATAL MR 18 MONTHS, AXIAL

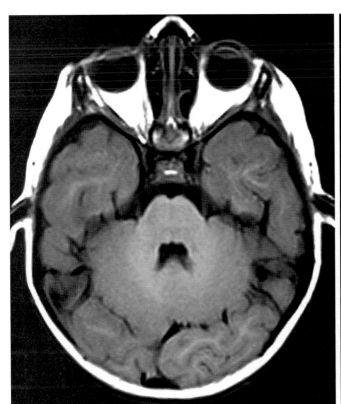
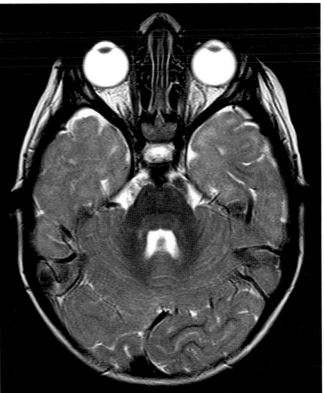

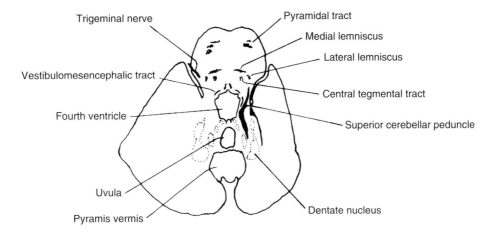

Trigeminal nerve

Pyramidal tract

Medial lemniscus

Lateral lemniscus

Vestibulomesencephalic tract

Central tegmental tract

Fourth ventricle

Superior cerebellar peduncle

Uvula

Dentate nucleus

Pyramis vermis

POSTNATAL MR 18 MONTHS, AXIAL

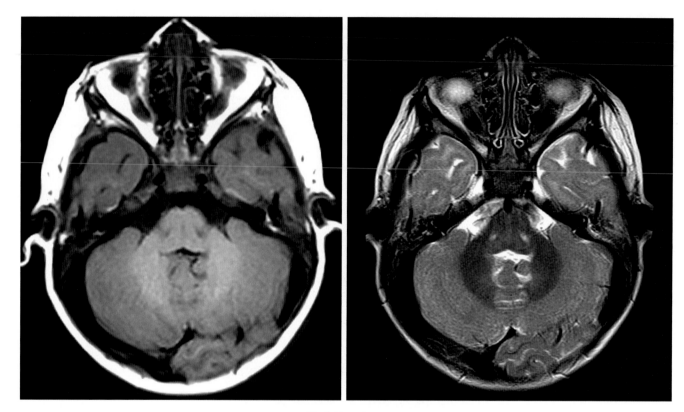

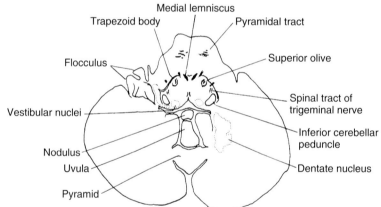

Medial lemniscus

Trapezoid body   Pyramidal tract

Flocculus   Superior olive

Vestibular nuclei   Spinal tract of
                                    trigeminal nerve

                                    Inferior cerebellar
Nodulus   peduncle

Uvula   Dentate nucleus

Pyramid

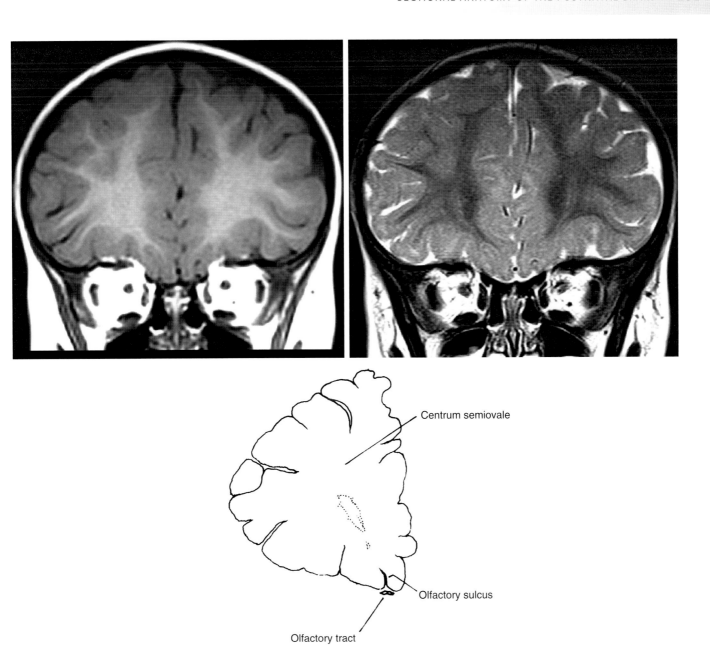

Centrum semiovale

Olfactory sulcus

Olfactory tract

POSTNATAL MR 18 MONTHS, CORONAL

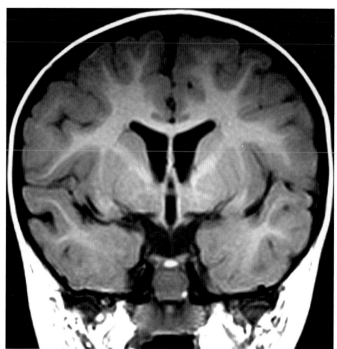
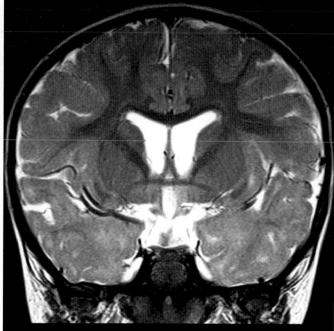

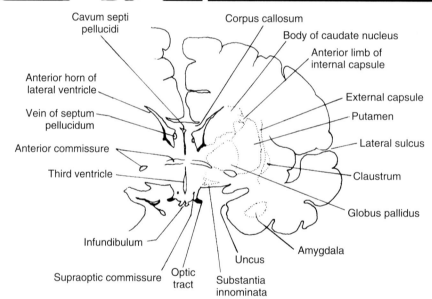

Cavum septi pellucidi

Corpus callosum

Body of caudate nucleus

Anterior limb of internal capsule

Anterior horn of lateral ventricle

External capsule

Vein of septum pellucidum

Putamen

Anterior commissure

Lateral sulcus

Third ventricle

Claustrum

Globus pallidus

Infundibulum

Amygdala

Supraoptic commissure

Optic tract

Uncus

Substantia innominata

POSTNATAL MR 18 MONTHS, CORONAL

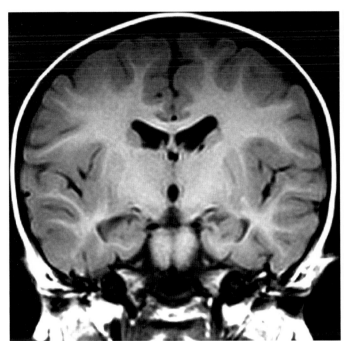
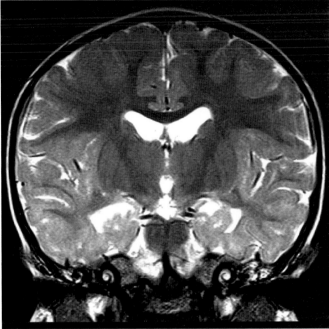

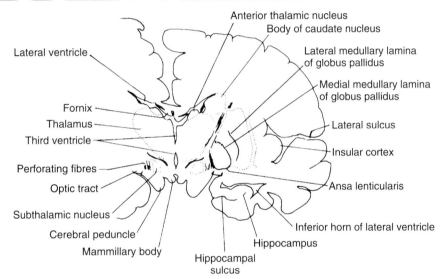

Anterior thalamic nucleus
Body of caudate nucleus
Lateral medullary lamina of globus pallidus
Medial medullary lamina of globus pallidus
Lateral sulcus
Insular cortex
Ansa lenticularis
Inferior horn of lateral ventricle
Lateral ventricle
Fornix
Thalamus
Third ventricle
Perforating fibres
Optic tract
Subthalamic nucleus
Cerebral peduncle
Mammillary body
Hippocampal sulcus
Hippocampus

POSTNATAL MR 18 MONTHS, CORONAL

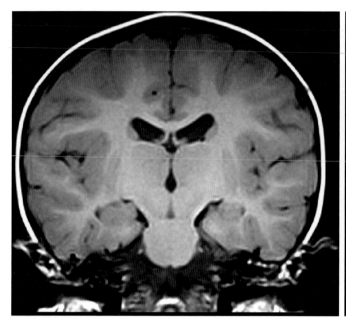
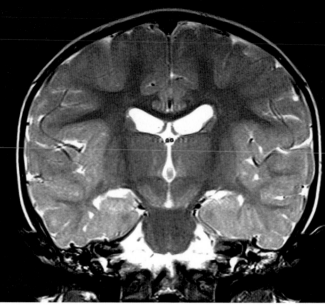

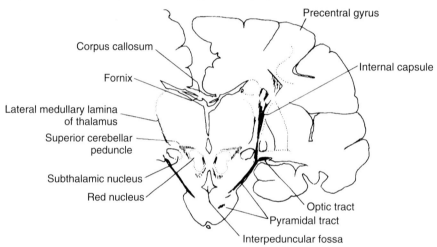

Precentral gyrus

Corpus callosum

Fornix

Internal capsule

Lateral medullary lamina
of thalamus

Superior cerebellar
peduncle

Subthalamic nucleus

Red nucleus

Optic tract

Pyramidal tract

Interpeduncular fossa

POSTNATAL MR 18 MONTHS, CORONAL

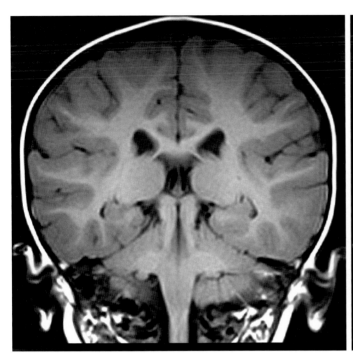
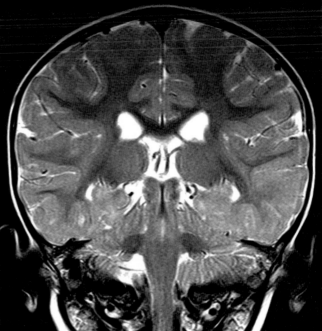

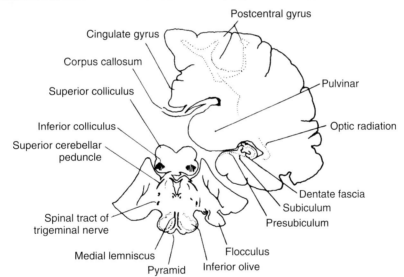

Cingulate gyrus

Corpus callosum

Superior colliculus

Inferior colliculus

Superior cerebellar peduncle

Spinal tract of trigeminal nerve

Medial lemniscus

Pyramid

Postcentral gyrus

Pulvinar

Optic radiation

Dentate fascia

Subiculum

Presubiculum

Flocculus

Inferior olive

POSTNATAL MR 18 MONTHS, CORONAL

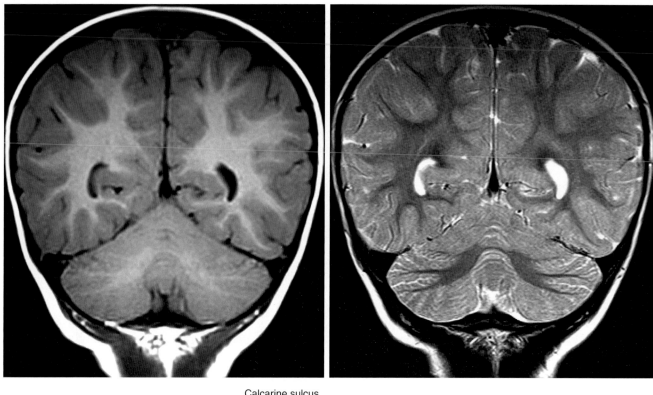

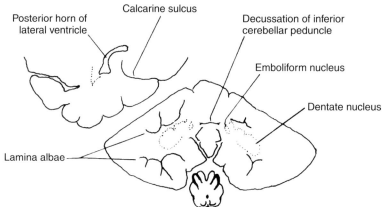

Posterior horn of
lateral ventricle

Calcarine sulcus

Decussation of inferior
cerebellar peduncle

Emboliform nucleus

Dentate nucleus

Lamina albae

POSTNATAL MR 18 MONTHS, CORONAL

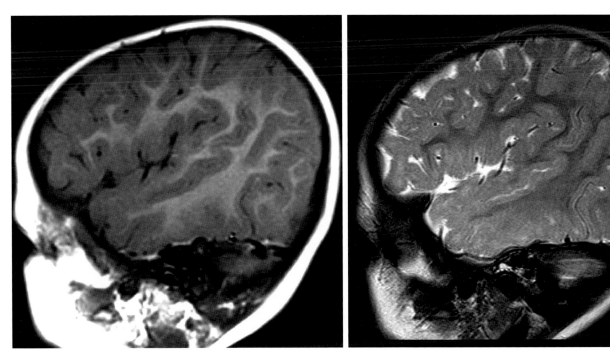

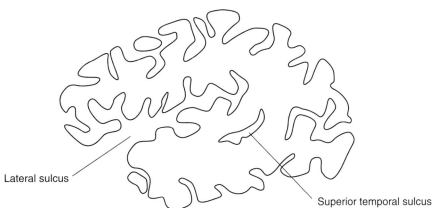

Lateral sulcus

Superior temporal sulcus

POSTNATAL MR 18 MONTHS, SAGITTAL

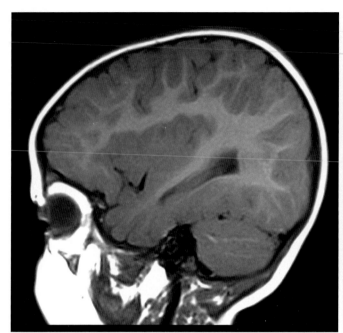
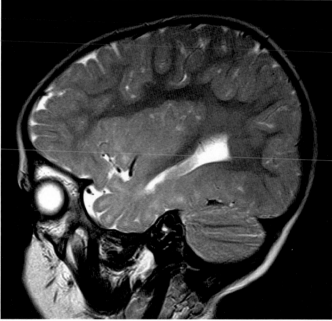

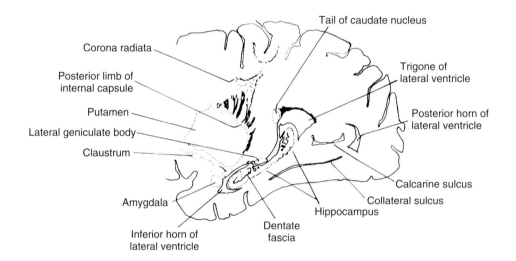

Corona radiata

Posterior limb of
internal capsule

Putamen

Lateral geniculate body

Claustrum

Amygdala

Inferior horn of
lateral ventricle

Dentate
fascia

Hippocampus

Tail of caudate nucleus

Trigone of
lateral ventricle

Posterior horn of
lateral ventricle

Calcarine sulcus

Collateral sulcus

POSTNATAL MR 18 MONTHS, SAGITTAL

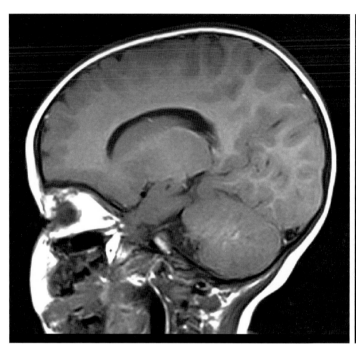
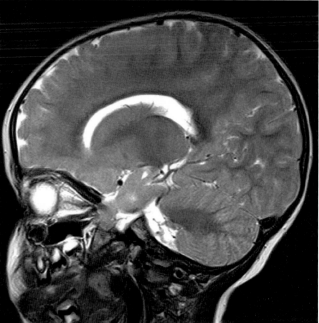

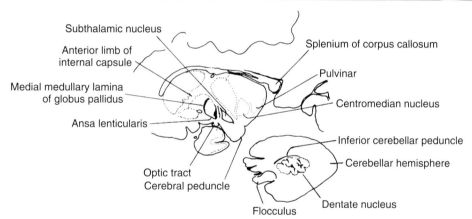

Subthalamic nucleus

Anterior limb of
internal capsule

Medial medullary lamina
of globus pallidus

Ansa lenticularis

Optic tract
Cerebral peduncle

Splenium of corpus callosum

Pulvinar

Centromedian nucleus

Inferior cerebellar peduncle

Cerebellar hemisphere

Dentate nucleus

Flocculus

POSTNATAL MR 18 MONTHS, SAGITTAL

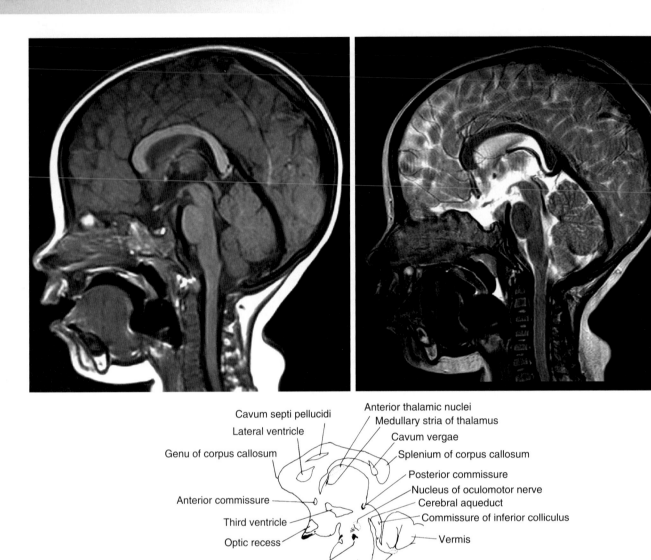

Cavum septi pellucidi

Lateral ventricle

Genu of corpus callosum

Anterior commissure

Third ventricle

Optic recess

Decussation of superior
cerebellar peduncle

Medial lemniscus

Pyramidal decussation

Anterior thalamic nuclei

Medullary stria of thalamus

Cavum vergae

Splenium of corpus callosum

Posterior commissure

Nucleus of oculomotor nerve

Cerebral aqueduct

Commissure of inferior colliculus

Vermis

Gracile nucleus

Cuneate nucleus

POSTNATAL MR 18 MONTHS, SAGITTAL